Theory and Nursing
a systematic approach

Theory and Nursing
a systematic approach

Peggy L. Chinn, RN, PhD, FAAN

Professor of Nursing and Associate Dean for Academics,
University of Colorado Health Sciences Center School of Nursing,
Denver, Colorado

Maeona K. Kramer, RN, PhD

Professor of Nursing,
University of Utah,
Salt Lake City, Utah

FOURTH EDITION

with 24 illustrations

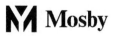 Mosby

St. Louis Baltimore Berlin Boston Carlsbad Chicago London Madrid
Naples New York Philadelphia Sydney Tokyo Toronto

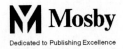

Senior Vice President, Editorial: Alison Harrison
Publisher: Nancy L. Coon
Managing Editor: Loren Stevenson Wilson
Associate Developmental Editor: Brian Dennison
Project Manager: Mark Spann
Production Editor: Stephen C. Hetager
Designer: David Zielinski
Manufacturing Supervisor: Karen Lewis

Fourth Edition

Printed in the United States of America

Composition by Shepherd, Inc.

Printing/binding by Wm. C. Brown Communications

Mosby-Year Book, Inc.
11830 Westline Industrial Drive
St. Louis, Missouri 63146

ISBN 0-8016-7947-8

95 96 97 98 99 / 9 8 7 6 5 4 3 2 1

Preface

Books, and revisions of books, reflect the trends of the time in which the book was conceived and written. This fourth edition is no exception. The end of the 1980s marked a growing emphasis in the nursing scholarly community on the need for *midrange theory*—theory that is more closely linked to the needs and demands of nursing practice. As we examined previous editions of this book, we realized that from the beginning we had emphasized the need for a practice-theory link, and had included information about midrange theory in nursing. However, until this edition, the nursing literature did not yet contain a substantial collection of midrange theory. This fourth edition of the book includes additional emphasis on the development of midrange theory in nursing, as well as specific examples from the nursing literature.

THE FOURTH EDITION

In addition to the changes related to midrange theory, we have made structural and content revisions throughout. The revisions that characterize this fourth edition are described in the following paragraphs:

Chapter 1 focuses on nursing's patterns of knowing. This chapter is intended to provide a general understanding of the nature of the whole of nursing knowledge, with empiric/scientific theory constituting a major part of one pattern. We have expanded our discussion of the methodologic approaches to developing knowledge within each of the patterns of knowing in nursing to show more clearly how the various patterns interrelate to form the whole of knowing.

Chapter 2 focuses on theory as the expression of empirics. We have retained the model for theory development that we used in prior editions of the book, but with the significant changes in language that we used to characterize theory development processes (see Notations on Language later in this preface). The model serves to emphasize the fact that several different, yet interdependent, types of activities are needed for the development of knowledge in a practice discipline.

Chapter 3 focuses on the historic emergence of the key concepts of the discipline. We have added the evolution of midrange practice-linked theory as a continuing process in the development of theory in nursing. We show a chronology of the evolving directions in theory during the first 40 years of formal theory development in nursing, continuing through the 1980s. We emphasize the shifts that emerged in the 1980s when nurse scholars began to focus on the development of research and theory at a midrange level, more specifically addressing problems and phenomena that are located within nursing's scope of practice and the health and illness experience of people who receive nursing care.

Chapter 4 reflects the shifts that have emerged in nursing concerning what types of theory and philosophy or ethic are required for practice. Our definition of theory is "a creative and rigorous structuring of ideas that project a tentative, purposeful, and systematic view of phenomena." A dramatic difference between our definition of theory and other definitions is the move away from the teleologic (outcome-focused) purposes of traditional science (description, explanation, and prediction). Our definition places the theorist at the center; it defines theory in a way that the theorist's own creativity is central in structuring a particular view stated as theory. This definition also moves toward a clearer differentiation between more global frameworks or models, and the more precisely focused midrange theories.

Chapter 5 fills in the details of how the various components of the processes for theory development emerge. In this edition we have expanded our consideration of how conceptual meaning is formed, and illustrate how additional data sources can contribute to the formation of conceptual meaning, particularly in the arts. The emphasis in this chapter is to convey approaches that you can use to truly create—to bring forth that which is useful for your research and practice purposes.

Chapters 6 and 7 focus on description (Chapter 6) and critical reflection (Chapter 7) of theory. Chapters 8 and 9 examine links between theory, research, and practice. We have updated these chapters to be consistent with our shift in focus to include midrange nursing theory.

We have retained the appendix that appeared in the previous edition (Appendix A), which consists of a brief overview of the work of nurse theorists whose work broadly defines nursing, and have added to this appendix the work of Patricia Benner and Judith Wrubel. We have added an appendix that provides overviews of selected midrange nursing theories (Appendix B), providing examples of recently emerging practice-specific areas of midrange theory. In preparing these overviews, we used the elements of our proposed model for theory development to show how these activities do indeed contribute to development of theory in a practice discipline. Finally, we have retained and updated the glossary, which provides definitions of key terms that we use in this book, as well as page references to discussions in the text.

NOTATIONS ON LANGUAGE*

Beginning with the third edition, we made profound shifts in the language of this book. The changes in language came from our growing awareness of both

---

*We acknowledge with gratitude the important influence and assistance of Charlene Eldridge Wheeler (1944-1993), who provided editorial and linguistic assistance with the third edition.

subtle and blatant meanings that contradicted the values that we held personally, and also values of nursing. Since these language changes and their inherent value shifts are not easily recognized, we include here the notations on the deliberate language changes that first appeared in the third edition.

Our initial aim with respect to changing the language of this book was to shift the writing style to a clearer, more accessible, and more readable form. We have always maintained as a basic premise of the book that theory, research, and practice need to "connect" with one another, and that nurses who work in academics and in practice need to be able to better communicate with one another. Consistent with this commitment we began the editing process with the intent to eliminate words and phrases that depended on or assumed a style typically reserved for the academician. We began by simplifying the sentence structure, eliminating pretentious words when a common word would do, shifting to the active voice as much as possible, and limiting the use of pronouns to instances when an agent is clearly identifiable.

As we worked, we became aware of more "flaws" in the underlying structure of the language and tried to address them as consistently as possible. We became conscious of value assumptions and connotations that were inherent in the language. Many of the terms that are commonly associated with the practice of scientific methods carry antagonistic, adversarial, objectifying, and militaristic connotations that are contrary to the intents of an ethic of caring and of human science. The term "whip lines" (now wave lines) is an example of a term that was built into our conception of the system for theory development. Other terms that we found to occur with impressive frequency were "competing images," "judgments," "capture," "aim," "target," "operation," "boundaries," "argument," and "debate." Even when the strict meaning of a word was adequate for the text, we sought to shift the language to words that carry a similar literal meaning but a more human and caring value connotation. For example, instead of the phrase "argue your position," we use instead "share your ideas."

There were other subtle meanings that we had built into the language and structure of earlier editions of the book, some of which were contradictory to our intent, an intent that dated back to the first edition. We did not intend to prescribe "set" or "best" metatheoretical approaches or to convey a strict adherence to linearity. Yet the semantic structure of much of what we presented resulted in an approach that was both prescriptive and linear. For example, in the third edition we shifted from a prescriptive criteria-based approach to theory description and evaluation, to a mode of questioning and considering alternatives. We have refined and enhanced this approach in this fourth edition, inviting you, the reader, to explore responses to the questions, forming avenues for creating new directions. We deleted references to the "first," "second," or "third" "step" in a process, speaking instead of issues or alternatives that could be addressed in the context of a process.

Another shift that we made in the language is informed by our intent to reframe traditional relationships between people. We have sought to directly engage and empower the reader. We speak directly to the reader as "you," with the intent to encourage the reader's own abilities and ideas rather than to impose the authoritative voice of the text. For example, in Chapter 5 we speak of how model cases are used in forming conceptual meaning by stating: "When you consider your model case placed in several different social contexts, you create an avenue for perceiving important values and make deliberate choices concerning them."

The language shifts that we have made lead to a profound difference in how we think about the processes for developing knowledge. We invite you to join us in a continual process of growing awareness of ways in which language creates and shapes our collective values, knowledge, and indeed, reality.

ACKNOWLEDGEMENTS

When we first conceived of the essential elements of this book, we had both recently completed our doctoral educations, and were entering our academic careers. We have both now entered our third decade of teaching. Individuals who have enrolled in our classes at all levels remain those to whom we owe our greatest debt of gratitude. Without your continual prodding for clearer explanations, your insistence in pushing us beyond the limits of our own preconceived notions, many of the ideas that have emerged in this book would not have been possible. Our many academic colleagues, both within the institutions where we have taught, and around the world, have contributed to our thinking by being our most informed, critical, and thoughtful audience. Our close friends and chosen families have continued to provide the love and support that are so essential to this type of work. As much as we feel deeply the ways in which this work depends on our interactions in all of these domains, we acknowledge that the content of this book remains our own doing and our own responsibility. We continue to provide for one another the challenges that are inherent in cowriting a work of this type, and the mutual respect and appreciation that sustain this type of relationship over time. We offer this work as a gift to our many colleagues and students in the hope that it will continue to provide a perspective that contributes to your understanding, and that inspires your own thinking and action.

Peggy L. Chinn
Maeona K. Kramer

Contents in Brief

Contents

CHAPTER 6   DESCRIPTION OF NURSING THEORY, 105

CHAPTER 7   CRITICAL REFLECTION OF NURSING THEORY, 125

1

Nursing's patterns of knowing

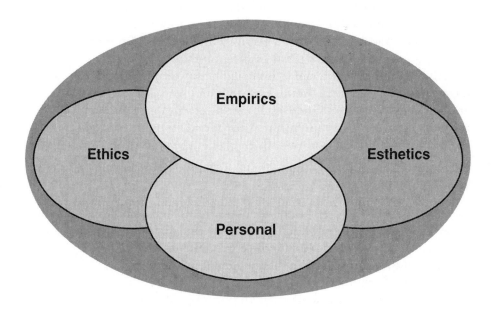

Empiric knowledge is part of a larger whole of knowing.
Each of the patterns of knowing is essential. Each is a
distinct aspect of the whole, every pattern makes a
contribution to the whole, and each is equally vital.
This chapter presents a conception of the whole
of knowing in nursing to show the unique aspects of each
component and provides the foundation for
understanding theory as expression of empiric knowledge.

ex. Mildred, pt CA colon

Since Nightingale first established formal education for nurses, nursing has depended on formal knowledge as a basis for practice. The type of knowledge seen as valuable in nursing has changed over the decades since Nightingale. Before 1950, nursing was viewed as a technical art that emphasized principles and procedures coupled with a spirit of unselfish devotion. By the 1950s, the phrase "nursing science" began to appear in the nursing literature. Today, nursing theory and research are seen as important means of achieving scientific knowledge for nursing practice.

Although nursing science is a valuable basis for nursing practice, knowledge that does not fit the traditional definition of science is also necessary and valuable. This chapter addresses the various forms of knowing on which nursing practice is based and provides the foundation for understanding theory as an expression of empirics, which is one type of nursing knowledge.

HOW DO WE KNOW?

The processes of knowing are common and fundamental human activities. Everyone, from the time of birth, begins a lifelong process of learning, of experiencing self, other people, and the environment. What people know is the outcome of these everyday experiences.

Processes for knowing in Western academic cultures have also been structured, formalized, and systematized. For example, Western scientists claim to know something because they have applied a particular research method or used a scientific problem-solving approach. Some nurses are educated and trained to use formalized approaches to produce structured knowledge that is known as a body of knowledge. These nurses who are engaged in producing new nursing knowledge collectively constitute and develop the discipline of nursing. Nurses who work in a nursing practice situation bring knowledge from lifelong experiences, as well as the structured knowledge of the discipline taught through education and training.

Although various ways of knowing have been acknowledged and described in Western societies, traditional science has acquired the status of a superior way for a group to develop knowledge and to establish what is thought of as truth. For example, Kerlinger (1986) identifies tenacity, authority, and a priori methods as ways of knowing that are inferior to science. According to this view, tenacity is the form of knowing in which the person believes that something is true without reason to question. Authority is a belief that something is true because an authoritative source or person says it is true. A priori knowing depends on reason and is not necessarily consistent with experience. Each of these forms of knowing can lead to the same conclusion about what is true. The difference between them is in *how* one knows. For example, some people might say that sitting in a draft causes a cold. If asked how they know this is so, they might state that it is just true (tenacity), that their parents told them so (authority), or that it stands to reason (a priori).

Knowledge about how a cold is transmitted may also be learned from the method of science. The method of science is different from tenacity, authority, or a priori ways of knowing in that empiric (experiential or sensory) evidence is used as the test of whether or not something is true. The methods of science were developed as a way to eliminate errors in judging what is true by repeated tests of hypotheses on the basis of empiric reality. From a traditional scientific perspective, only what stands the test of repeated empiric testing constitutes knowledge, or truth. Therefore, if someone decided to examine whether sitting in a draft causes colds, this idea would be stated as a hypothesis and repeatedly tested to determine if empiric evidence supported the claim.

All of the forms of knowing described by Kerlinger rest on an idea about objectivity in which truth is thought to exist apart from, or outside of, the person who knows. A fundamental idea about reality from which traditional science developed is Descartian dualism, in which the rational mind and the "out there" reality of truth are viewed as separate.

A shift in ideas about the value of science as a superior way to know is emerging in nursing and society. These emerging ideas are based on a view that assumes a fundamental unity between the knower and what is known (Bleich, 1978). From this perspective, the person who perceives reality is recognized as an active participant in creating what is known. The assumption is that knowledge is created by people and not objectively discovered as an "out there" reality. The emphasis is on making sense of the world in terms of the needs of the present and the future, on resolving the splits and contradictions that the traditional objective methods cannot resolve, and on seeking tentative understandings rather than absolute truth (Chinn, 1985).

The term *human science* has evolved in the social sciences and is used in nursing to refer to processes for empiric inquiry that account for and respect human characteristics such as motivation and intentionality. Human science methods acknowledge the effect of the scientist on what is studied. They are designed to account for the changing nature of human experience and the role of choice and meaning in determining human action (Polkinghorne, 1983).

While working with people who have health problems, nurses are constantly reminded of the reality that mind and body are a unity. Any one experience reflects and will be reflected in the whole. Individuals with whom nurses interact are not only cells, body organs, or minds, but people with all of these dynamic traits who have families and cultures, past histories, and futures. All people have personal values and beliefs that have undeniable influence on experiences of health and illness.

Nurses also recognize the unrealistic split between theory and practice. Nurse scholars, educators, and practitioners have urged the building of bridges between what we know and what we do in practice (Benner and Wrubel, 1989). Theory that has practice value will not emerge exclusively from the methods of science. Theory that draws on multiple patterns of knowing will provide a valuable link between the worlds of practice and theory so they are not perceived as separate.

We believe that a hierarchic distinction between ways of knowing is not useful as an approach to developing nursing knowledge. Not only does this view place science in a superior position to other forms of knowing, but it overlooks forms of knowing that are valuable and necessary, even though different in form from science. In this text, we view knowing, knowledge, and the development of knowledge from a holistic perspective in that no single form of knowledge or way of knowing is judged to be superior or inferior to any other form. Different ways of knowing are not judged against one another. Rather, different ways of knowing and of creating knowledge are each, in their own right, useful for some purpose. Science is well suited for some purposes but not for others. Nurses routinely encounter situations that require decisions and actions for which there are no scientific answers. In many of these situations, other forms of knowing provide insight and understanding. For example, ethical problems require methods that are suitable for addressing human values of rights and responsibilities.

Carper (1978) examined nursing literature and described four patterns of knowing that nurses have valued and used in practice: (1) ethics, the component of moral knowledge in nursing; (2) esthetics, the art of nursing; (3) personal knowing in nursing; and (4) empirics, the science of nursing. Each of the patterns of knowing described by Carper is equally necessary with each pattern contributing an essential component for the practice of nursing. Taken together, the patterns provide a basis for developing comprehensive knowledge. The following sections of this chapter present a conceptualization of how knowledge can be developed in nursing by drawing on Carper's four patterns of knowing.

THE WHOLE OF KNOWING

Nursing's patterns of knowing are interrelated processes that arise from the whole of experience. Informal, common, or everyday forms of knowing, as well as more formal ways of developing knowledge, contribute to useful knowledge for a practice discipline. In this text, we use the term *knowing* to refer to the individual human processes of experiencing and comprehending the self and the world in ways that can be brought to some level of conscious awareness. Knowing is a dynamic, changing process. We use the term *knowledge* to refer to what can be shared or communicated with others. Some forms in which knowledge is communicated are words or other symbols, actions, art, or sounds. Once expressed, knowledge can be passed along to others and can enter another person's conscious awareness.

Each of the patterns of knowing is an aspect of the whole. Every pattern makes a unique contribution to the whole of knowing, and each is equally vital. Each pattern describes something about the whole of nursing knowledge. This construction of knowing provides a way to think about the purpose, expression, and processes for development of knowledge in nursing. However, the patterns exist only as dimensions of the whole of knowing in nursing and cannot be used separately from the whole. For example, an ethical problem in practice might be addressed at the outset using methods of dialogue and justification. As the situation unfolds in practice, aspects of empirics, personal knowing, and esthetics will also find expression, usually in synchrony with one another. The academic exercise of attempting to separate one pattern from another refines ways of thinking and methods that contribute to an integrated process.

Figure 1–1 is a representation of the whole of knowing based on each of the patterns originally described by Carper. In the figure, each shaded area represents a distinct pattern—ethics, esthetics, personal, and empirics—

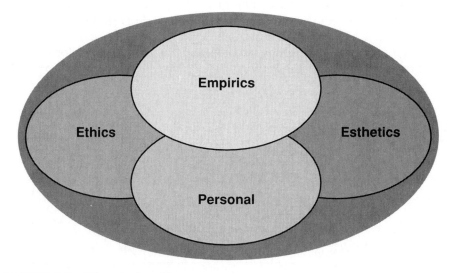

FIGURE 1–1   The whole of knowing.

within the whole of knowing. Considering each pattern of the whole is like viewing a portion of the sky with a telescope; the telescope enlarges and brings into focus a distinct portion of the universe, but the viewer can also step away from the telescope and perceive the whole sky. Perception of each portion is influenced by the perception of the whole, and perception of the whole is also influenced by the ability to perceive each portion more clearly through the telescope.

Some form of expression is needed for each pattern so that what is created can be communicated and so that the discipline can agree on methods for developing knowledge (Jacobs-Kramer and Chinn, 1988). As nurses practice, they know more than they can communicate. Some of what is known in practice can be expressed in words, actions, movements, or sounds, but much of what is known cannot be fully expressed. Attempting to express knowledge helps nurses focus, shape, influence, and communicate what is experienced. Expression makes it possible to move into a community, beyond the isolation of individual experience. Once this begins to happen, social purposes can form, and knowledge that helps the group to achieve its purposes can be shared. The process of developing shared knowledge opens possibilities for choices in nursing practice. The whole of knowing makes it possible to perceive what is possible and to create alternatives on which conscious choices can be made.

In Table 1–1, the creative and expressive dimensions of each pattern are described. The creative dimensions involve drawing on experience and making sense of that experience to move toward what can be or might be in the future. The expressive dimensions involve human actions—words, behaviors, and other symbols—that give communicable form to what we know and are not the same as what is known. The creative dimensions are human activities

TABLE 1–1 Patterns of knowing: creative and expressive dimensions

Dimension	Empiric	Ethics	Personal	Esthetics
Creative	Describing	Valuing	Opening	Engaging
	↕	↕	↕	↕
	Explaining	Clarifying	Centering	Intuiting
	↕	↕	↕	↕
	Predicting	Advocating	Realizing	Envisioning
Expressive	Facts, models, theories, and descriptions	Ethical theory, principles, and guidelines	Authentic genuine self	Art/Act

that individuals can pursue alone or can work in concert with others who share a common interest. Creative activities or processes are required to form the expressions that convey to others what is understood or known. Two of the patterns of knowing—ethics and empirics—are expressed in familiar forms of language. The expression of the patterns of esthetics and personal knowing is human actions and behavior rather than words. These human actions are also familiar, but they are commonly seen as expressions of personality or art, not as expressions of human knowing (Jacobs-Kramer and Chinn, 1988).

The traditions of science rest on the assumption that knowledge exists only to the extent that it can be objectified. Linguistic and mathematic forms of expression are the ideal in the scientific tradition. But, as the limits of empirics have become increasingly evident, it has become apparent that not all knowing can be communicated in language, and, in fact, language may distort the richness of human experience. Some form of communication is required for mutual understanding among people, but, because of its highly abstract nature, language also confounds shared understanding. As valuable and necessary as language is, it is not the only form of communication or expression that is available for human interaction. As other forms of expression come to be recognized and valued for their contribution to knowing processes, knowledge will become more whole and complete.

Empirics: the science of nursing

Empirics as the science of nursing emerged as a concept in nursing during the late 1950s (Carper, 1978). Empirics as a pattern of knowing draws on traditional ideas of science in which reality is viewed as something that can be verified by other observers. Empirics is based on the assumption that what is known is accessible through the senses—seeing, touching, hearing, and so forth. The development of empiric knowledge has traditionally been accomplished by the methods of scientific hypothesis testing. Although most conceptualizations of empiric knowledge in nursing are linked to this traditional view of science, ideas about what is legitimate for the science of nursing have broadened to include activities that are not strictly within the realm of hypothesis testing, such as phenomenological descriptions or inductive (grounded) means of generating theory.

The processes related to creating empiric knowledge are describing, explaining, or predicting (see Table 1–1). A discipline focuses on a specific area of inquiry to predict, explain, or describe those things that are central to its purpose. Observations based on experience, facts, and impressions are expressed as organized descriptions. Empiric knowing may also be expressed as conceptual models and theories that explain and predict relationships. These formally constructed ideas form what is commonly identified as a body of knowledge.

Many of nursing's theories, conceptual models, and research efforts re-flect an ideal of scientific inquiry. Nursing theories have been judged against the ideals of scientific theory. However, many traits of theories in general—and nursing theories in particular—both draw on and reflect other patterns of knowing besides empirics.

The ideal of scientific theory requires that all the major ideas of a theory be expressed in terms that can be translated to "out there" empiric reality. According to this ideal, if a theory addresses an idea of health, definitions of health should point to the specific behavior or traits that can be measured or at least inferred as representative of health. For example, if one of these traits is blood pressure, the theory suggests which blood pressure values should be present to represent health. Nursing theorists have included specific observable traits and behaviors related to their ideas of health, but their writings also reflect the influence of individual values and beliefs regarding ideas such as health. Nursing theorists have also addressed the person of the nurse and the people with whom nurses interact, as well as insights that arise from the art of nursing. These dimensions of experience cannot be reduced to specific and measurable traits; thus, patterns of knowing other than empirics are embedded in existing theories of nursing. As a result, when theories of nursing are judged against traditional ideals of science, nursing theories are recognizably different from the ideal. However, in our view, nursing theories have traits that are consistent with the ideals of traditional science, but because other patterns of knowing are also embedded in them, they assume a significance that moves beyond the limits of traditional science. In this text, we focus on the development of theory that expresses empiric knowing as a component of the whole rather than as simply the component of empirics.

Ethics: moral knowledge in nursing

Ethics in nursing are focused on matters of obligation or what ought to be done. The moral component of knowing in nursing goes beyond mere knowledge of the norms or ethical codes of nursing, other related disciplines, and society; it involves making moment-to-moment judgments about what should be done, what is good and right, and what is responsible. Making ethical judgments often involves confronting conflicting values, norms, interests, or principles. There may be no satisfactory answer to an ethical dilemma—only imperfect alternatives, none of which are satisfactory. Ethical knowing in nursing requires both an implicit knowledge on which difficult on-the-spot decisions are based and knowledge of the formal principles and ethical theories of the discipline and society (Carper, 1978).

Creative processes of ethical knowing in nursing are clarifying, valuing, and advocating. The processes of valuing and clarifying explicate different philosophic positions about what is good, what is right, whose interest is being served, which actions are responsible, and what the goals are of those actions. Clarifying and valuing form the foundation for a personal ethic. These processes are used when nurses serve as advocates for the rights and responsibilities of others, as well as themselves.

The creative processes yield the expressive forms of ethical theory, ethical principles, and ethical guidelines. These forms of expression set forth the philosophic ideas on which ethical decisions rest. Ethical knowledge does not describe or prescribe what a decision should be; rather, it provides insight about which choices are possible and why. Ethical theories are like empiric theories in that they can describe some dimensions of reality and can express relationships between phenomena. However, empiric theory relies on explicit reference to observable reality to be tested. Ethical theory cannot be tested in this sense, because the relationships of the theory rest on underlying philosophic reasoning that cannot be empirically known. Empiric research can provide information and facts to guide the development of ethical knowledge and to assist in forming sound ethical decisions. However, empiric methods cannot be used to test ethical theory.

Personal knowing in nursing

Personal knowing in nursing concerns the inner experience of becoming a whole, aware self. As Carper (1978, p. 18) states, "One does not know about the self, one strives simply to know the self." It is through knowing the self that one is able to know another human being as a person. Personal knowing can encompass spiritual or metaphysical forms of knowing. Full awareness of the self, the moment, and the context of interaction makes possible meaningful, shared human experience. Without this component of knowing, the idea of "therapeutic use of self" in nursing would not be possible (Carper, 1978).

The creative processes of personal knowing are opening, centering, and realizing. Opening involves taking in the fullness of experience with conscious awareness. Centering is the process of contemplation and introspection that forms inner personal meaning from life experiences. Realizing is a process of expressing through personality, behavior, words, and deeds the genuine, real, whole self that is consistent with what is experienced in the inner life.

Unlike empirics and ethics, personal knowing is not directly expressed in language. The self is only fully communicated or described as the existence of self. What is perceived by others *is* the existence of the person or personality— the self. As personal knowing emerges more fully throughout life, the unique or genuine self can be more fully expressed and becomes accessible as a means by which deliberate action and interaction take form. Although personal knowledge is not directly communicable in words, it is possible to describe certain things about the self. Self-description is important in creating a shared understanding of how personal knowledge can be developed and used in a deliberative way. Descriptions about the self are limited in that they never fully reflect personal knowing, and they are retrospective in that they can only describe the self that was. However, descriptions can be a tool for developing self-awareness and self-intimacy and for communicating to others valuable ways of developing personal knowing (Hagan, 1990).

Esthetics: the art of nursing

Esthetic knowing in nursing is the comprehension of meaning in a singular, particular, subjective expression that we call the art/act. Esthetic knowing makes it possible to move beyond the limits and circumstances of a particular moment, to sense the meaning of the moment, and to envision what is possible but not yet real. Esthetic knowing in nursing is made visible through the actions, bearing, conduct, attitudes, and interactions of the nurse in response to others. Esthetic knowing is what makes possible knowing what to do with the moment, instantly, without conscious deliberation. It can also transform the immediate encounter into a direct perception of what is significant in it— that is, knowing or imparting meaning to what is being expressed in the encounter. Perception of meaning in an immediate encounter is what creates an artful nursing action, and the nurse's perception of meaning is reflected in the action taken (Carper, 1978).

Esthetic knowing involves the creative processes of engaging, intuiting,[1] and envisioning. Engaging is a direct involvement of the self within a situation. The experience does not depend on mental structures or cognitive representations or explanations. Rather, the meaning of the moment comes from deep within the subjective experience, is intuited from the context of the individual's human experiences, and becomes expressed through in-the-moment being in the situation, Intuiting leads directly to creative responses to the unique meaning of the moment and envisioning of new creative possibilities. As esthetic knowing develops, the art/act of nursing emerges; that is, the nurse's actions take on the element of artistry, creating unique, meaningful, deeply moving interactions with others that touch common chords of human experience.

Like personal knowing, esthetics is not expressed in language but artistically in the moment of experience-action. We refer in this text to the expres-

---

[1]Our use of this concept is a departure from Carper's original conception of esthetic knowing and is based on recent work of Chinn (1994) and other works published in Chinn and Watson (Eds.) (1994).

sion of the art/act, because nursing's art form tends to be the artful ways in which nurses interact with people and perform skilled tasks (Benner, 1984; Benner and Wrubel, 1989). The possibility for using the mediums of cultural art forms such as music, dance, and poetry as expressions of esthetic knowing in nursing also exists and is beginning to be explored in nursing (Watson, 1988; Chinn and Watson, 1994).

Each art/act is a unique and particular instance that cannot be replicated; the creation of each art/act exists only in the moment. What is expressed as a work of art, an act, arises from and comprises the esthetic experience. As with personal knowing, knowledge about the processes and experiences of esthetics can be communicated retrospectively, and components of skills involved in esthetic knowing can be shared. For example, comforting someone in pain is a component of nursing behavior that often reflects esthetic knowing in nursing. Certain traits of comforting a person in pain can be communicated, and the behaviors associated with comforting can be learned. However, esthetic knowing is expressed directly in the art/act; it only occurs in the moment and is unique to the particular esthetic experience. What is shared in the art/act becomes part of shared understanding in the the discipline.

PROCESSES FOR FORMING UNDERSTANDING

Nursing's patterns of knowing provide ways for sharing insights and understanding that can be used in practice. By understanding, we mean integrated comprehension that includes taking in the significance, background meanings, facts, and experiences as a whole. Understanding implies taking a perspective regarding truth that is open and dynamic; understanding does not imply utter certainty. Understanding includes what is known in a personal sense and what is knowledge in a collective sense. It also implies bringing a critical perspective to what is known in order to create new insights and new knowledge. Each pattern of knowing has its own unique, distinct method for forming understanding. These methods are directly influenced by the creative and expressive dimensions of each of the patterns, but they also provide bridges for integrating the whole of knowing that is more than the sum of the parts.

Table 1–2 summarizes the processes for forming understanding. The processes for each pattern include critical questions that are addressed and social/political processes of interaction that bring knowledge into the collective realm of the discipline. The social/political process is composed of interactive methods that are carried out in relation to the expression of each pattern of knowing. These methods reflect traditions and philosophic foun-

TABLE 1–2   Patterns of knowing: processes for forming understanding

Processes	Empiric	Ethics	Personal	Esthetics
Critical question	What is this? How does it work?	Is this right? For whom? Is this responsible?	Do I know what I do? Do I do what I know?	What does this mean?
Social/political process	Replication ↕ Validation	Dialogue ↕ Justification	Response ↕ Reflection	Consensus ↕ Criticism

dations on which the pattern of knowing rests. The methods represent a form of human interaction whereby the individual and the group find a common ground for making sense of the world. We have called these methods and interactions a social/political process to convey that forming understanding depends on the totality of culturally acquired expectations for human interactions, the influence of the particular period of history, the trends of the time, the place, and the social order. The process of forming understanding begins with fundamental critical questions that reflect the nature of each pattern of knowing. The questions that we suggest here are not the only questions that might be posed, but they are representative of the basic questions that tend to direct the activities of inquiry arising from that pattern. Each pattern of knowing has its own style, its own variety and types of approaches, and its own perspective for judging the adequacy of the method itself. The social/political process makes it possible to integrate each of the patterns of knowing into a whole.

Replication and validation are the processes of empirics that contribute to understanding. Because of the familiarity of these processes in traditional science, replication and validation are sometimes mistakenly assumed to be appropriate as methods for other patterns of knowing. However, replication and validation are only useful for empirics. These processes require systematic empiric investigations that address such fundamental questions as "What is this?" and "How does it work?" Replication and validation require consistent agreement between people; what is thought to be for one person or context must hold true for another. Evidence related to an empiric theory is expected to be replicable in other times and situations to determine if the realities hold true even with changing circumstances.

The social/political process of the ethical pattern of knowing is dialogue and justification. Critical questions that are addressed in relation to this pat-

tern of knowing including "Is this right?" "For whom?" and "Is this responsible?" Ethical knowing does not require agreement in order to form understanding. Rather, ethical justification requires that fundamental value
assumptions are made explicit and that a line of reasoning emerges so that
others can follow the basis on which the individual reaches an ethical conclusion (theory, principles, guidelines). As ethical knowledge is expressed, dialogue becomes the social/political process so that the ideas are challenged,
rethought, reformed, and made clearer. This process makes it possible for a
group to examine carefully the ethical basis for actions with respect to the
group's collective and agreed-on purposes or intents.

Reflection and response are the processes of personal knowing that contribute to understanding. The critical question that is addressed is "Do I know
what I do, and do I do what I know?" Reflection requires the integration of a
wide range of information and understanding derived from all forms of knowing and from other knowers, and an internal accounting of how fully what is
known is actualized or realized within the self of the knower. Responses from
others mirror or reflect the ways the person is perceived. As the responses of
others are received, the individual gains insights that can be used in the self-
reflection process, and the self becomes, or is realized, as an authentic being
in the world.

Criticism and consensus are the social/political processes that contribute
to forming understanding in esthetics. A critical question that is asked within
this pattern of knowing is "What does this mean?" Criticism is a method that
reveals meanings; it focuses on creating insights that can move beyond what
is to something that might be in the future. *Criticism* is defined as "deliberate,
critical, precise, thoughtful reflection and action directed toward transformation" (Wheeler and Chinn, 1989, p. 37). The method of criticism as we envision it draws on criticism as used in the arts, where

> The art critic brings to the art insights and interpretations that help others to
> appreciate more fully what the artist has done, and what the art means for the
> culture as a whole. The critic does not proclaim the "correct" view of the art,
> but does provide a well-informed, knowledgeable interpretation of the art
> that helps others understand the art better, even if they don't agree with the
> views of the critic (Wheeler and Chinn, 1989, p. 37).

Rather than seeking agreement, esthetics depends on the process of consensus, where individuals bring to full awareness the diverse perspectives of
others in the group, comprehend the realities of those perspectives, and integrate knowledge of those perspectives. Consensus depends on an empathic
move that places each individual in the situation of the other, so that the perspective of the other can be fully appreciated. Out of this grows the capacity
for the artful, deeply human interactions that are central to nursing practice.

INTEGRATION

As Carper demonstrated in identifying the patterns of knowing, nursing has a long history of using various patterns. What has been missing is an explicit recognition of the value of all patterns of knowing as legitimate sources of collective nursing knowledge.

Ethical knowing has been recognized as necessary in an increasingly crowded, complex technologic society, but the empirically discernible factors that are associated with ethics have been valued above the philosophic methods that are needed to create new ethical knowledge in nursing. Likewise, personal knowing has been acknowledged as an important component of nursing practice in order to develop interpersonal relationships that are recognized as therapeutic. However, personal knowing has not been viewed as a legitimate or formal source of new knowledge. Like personal knowing, esthetics has been recognized as an important source of insight for nursing practice, but esthetics has not been explored or valued for its potential contribution to the development of new knowledge. Both personal knowing and esthetics have been kept private with little attention given to developing forms for their expression. Each pattern of knowing is distinct in its expression and its methods for contributing to understanding. Each pattern is equally necessary for full understanding, full knowing, and the development of a collective body of knowledge for nursing practice (Carper, 1978).

Figure 1–2 illustrates the interconnections between the creative processes and the social/political processes for determining credibility for each pat-

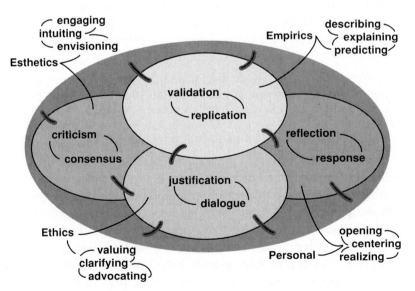

FIGURE 1–2   Interconnections of model processes.

tern. As processes for forming understanding are engaged, knowledge takes the form of an integrated whole. Each set of processes is distinct for individual patterns of knowing, but they draw on, and contribute to, the processes within the whole of the patterns of knowing.

Suppose you want to address an ethical question concerning what is right. You might begin with the focused creative activities of making explicit the personal and group values (valuing) that should guide your actions, clarifying the positions you find in ethical theories and principles that inform the issue, and setting forth (advocating) how the application of these principles would function with the people with whom you work. These processes would lead you to a justification of your ideas based primarily in ethical reasoning. When you begin to share your ideas with your colleagues (the social/political context), the questioning and discussion that results will bring to awareness the personal insights of others engaged in the dialogue, the empirical evidence about similar situations, and the range of esthetic meanings that are possible in this and similar situations.

If you have an empirical problem concerning what nursing action is most effective in practice, you might begin by designing research methods to describe the nature of a caring process, such as comforting. You would explain how comfort is achieved and predict the circumstances under which comfort emerges. In developing and implementing your program of research, you assess theories of comfort, developing your own evolving theory. As you move toward the social/political processes of validation and replication, your focus will expand to integrate esthetic meaning of experiences of comfort and of giving comfort, personal insight concerning the experience of comfort, and ethical values that influence how comfort is given and received.

Personal knowing is frequently the avenue through which awareness of possibilities that are not yet fully understood first emerges. For example, suppose a nurse has a growing uneasiness about a customary procedure in giving care. Something does not seem to fit, does not feel right, or does not make sense. When this sense grows, the nurse's awareness opens, and the nurse becomes sensitive to details of the situation that previously were taken for granted. The nurse centers on processes and contexts that help to make sense of the personal experience with the procedure, gradually developing realizations that become part of the nurse's understanding. When these personal insights are shared with others, collective reflection and response lead to explorations of other ways of knowing and understanding the experience of the procedure. As nurses share their personal insights, meanings, empiric evidence, and ethical issues, they form integrated understanding and knowing of the procedure. Out of this process, nurses can create changes in how things are done, in empiric research studies, or in artistic expressions that express deeper meanings of the situation.

Esthetics as a starting point, like personal knowing, often begins with a nurse's own awareness, but the expression takes an art form. The art can be in the form of the nurse's action in a situation. Suppose a nurse feels a connection to a person's experience of chronic pain. In a moment of caring for the person, the nurse acts from a deeply developed knowing of the meaning of chronic pain in a way that connects with the person's own experience. Or, the nurse might develop a story, create a painting, or compose a poem as an avenue to metaphorically represent the experience in ways that are not possible to express fully in any other form. Regardless of form, esthetics emerges through the processes of envisioning the experience of chronic pain, intuiting its meaning, and engaging with the artistic medium to create the expression. When the action, story, poem, or painting is shared, others take in the nurse's message, growing in awareness of both the unique and shared meanings of pain. The technical or empirical aspects of the art, the ethical aspects of what is represented, and the personal meanings are brought together in the form of criticism that conveys even fuller collective understanding of the human experience (Chinn and Watson, 1994).

PATTERNS GONE WILD

When knowledge within any one pattern is not critically examined and integrated with the whole of knowing, distortion instead of understanding is produced. Failure to integrate all of the patterns of knowing leads to uncritical acceptance, narrow interpretation, and partial utilization of knowledge. We call this "the patterns gone wild." When this occurs, the patterns are used in isolation from one another, and the potential for integration is lost.

Empirics removed from the context of the whole of knowing produces control and manipulation. Ironically, these have been explicit traditional goals of the empiric sciences. When the validity of empiric knowledge is not questioned, one danger is its potential use in contexts where it does not belong. When you recognize how all the patterns contribute to the validity of empirics, you begin to see the goals of control and manipulation as a distortion or misuse of empiric knowledge.

Ethics removed from the context of the whole of knowing produces rigid doctrine and insensitivity to the rights of others. This happens when someone simply sets forth her own ideas concerning what is right or good advocating her position on the reasoning derived from her own perspective. She may even present a justification for her perspective to others but does not take seriously the processes of dialogue that her justification invites. In the absence of this integrating process, her position remains isolated, with little or no opportunity for empirical, personal, or esthetic insights to give meaning and social relevance to her ideas.

Personal knowing removed from the context of the whole of knowing produces isolation and self-distortion. When this happens, the self remains isolated, and knowledge of self comes only from what is known internally. Self-distortions can take a wide range of forms, from aggrandizement and overestimation of self to destruction and underestimation of self.

Esthetics removed from the context of the whole of knowing produces prejudice, bigotry, and lack of appreciation for the fullness of meaning in a context. Human actions emerge from and are represented by the tastes and desires of the individual alone, without taking into account the deep cultural meanings inherent in the art/act. Art/acts become self-serving, shallow, arrogant, and empty. Preferences that reflect social prejudice and bigotry also grow out of a failure to comprehend the deeper cultural, historical, and political significance of an art/act. Unauthentic meanings are assigned to another's experience, or a self-serving posture is assumed with respect to another person.

To illustrate the "patterns gone wild," imagine an elderly woman admitted to a nursing home. She has lived a life rich in experience and activities and loves to verbally explore her past, making sense of what it means and how it relates to her present life. Having always been physically active, she takes a nightly stroll before going to bed. In the nursing home, she climbs over the bed rails after the lights are out, and, with her walker, walks the halls, unsteady but determined, smiling and peering into other rooms. Sometimes, hearing other residents talking or moaning, she goes into their room and tells them stories or talks with them to ease their troubled night.

Consider what you might see in a nursing care plan if any one of the patterns of knowing were isolated from the context of the whole of knowing. Empirics isolated from the other patterns of knowing might require giving a drug that would be effective in bringing sleep to the woman soon after the lights go out, thereby controlling the situation and manipulating her into compliance, regardless of any other concerns. Ethics taken alone might impose the nurse's view of what is right or good for the woman, leading to a rule that would punish the woman if she left her bed after the lights went out and creating a rigid, rule-oriented atmosphere that is insensitive to what the woman and others see as right or good. Personal knowing in isolation would impose the nurse's perspective without comprehending the meaning of the woman's experience for her, the empirical explanations of her behavior, or the ethics of caring. When this happens, the nurse remains isolated in the self-centered view that the old woman is a nuisance who is interfering with the time needed to complete the charting for the night. Esthetics alone would impose the nurse's own tastes, preferences, and meanings on the situation. When values, empirical knowledge, and personal sensitivities do not inform individual esthetic interpretations, situational meanings remain parochial.

The prejudiced idea that this experience has no cultural meaning, that old people are too ugly, frail, and feeble to wander around the halls, and that by doing so they might hurt themselves, can lead to restraining the woman or taking other action that is self-serving to the nurse.

When ethical, esthetic, personal knowing, and empirics are integrated, the purposes of developing knowledge and the actions based on that knowledge become more responsible and humane and create liberating choices.

CONCLUSION

In this chapter, we considered nursing's patterns of knowing and introduced ideas about how the whole of knowing emerges. We have described traits of each pattern—empiric, ethical, esthetic, and personal knowing. We introduced ideas about creative processes and forms of expressing knowledge that emerge from each of the patterns of knowing. There are methods suited to each pattern that can contribute to the process of forming understanding. The methods of personal knowing, ethics, and esthetics are introduced here and will be further developed in another text. In Chapter 2, we consider theory as an expression of empirics, which forms the focus for this book.

REFERENCES

Benner P: From novice to expert: excellence and power in cinical nursing practice, Menlo Park, 1984, Addison-Wesley.

Benner P and Wrubel J: The primacy of caring, Menlo Park, 1989, Addison-Wesley.

Bleich D: Subjective criticism, Baltimore, 1978, Johns Hopkins University Press.

Carper BA: Fundamental patterns of knowing in nursing, *Adv Nurs Sci* 1(1):13–23, 1978.

Chinn PL: Debunking myths in nursing theory and research, *Image* 17(2):45–49, 1985.

Chinn PL and Watson MJ: Anthology on art and aesthetics in nursing, New York, 1994, National League for Nursing.

Hagan KL: Internal affairs: a journalkeeping workbook for self-intimacy, New York, 1990, Harper & Row.

Jacobs-Kramer MK and Chinn PL: Perspectives on knowing: a model of nursing knowledge, *Scholarly Inquiry Nurs Pract* 2(2):129–39, 1988.

Kerlinger FN: Foundations of behavioral research, ed 3, New York, 1986, Holt, Rinehart & Winston, Inc.

Polkinghorne D: Methodology for the human sciences, Albany, 1983, SUNY Press.

Watson J: New dimensions of human caring theory, *Nurs Sci Q* 1(4):175–181, 1988.

Wheeler CE and Chinn PL: Peace and power: a handbook of feminist process, ed 3, New York, 1991, National League for Nursing.

2

Nursing theory as an expression of empirics

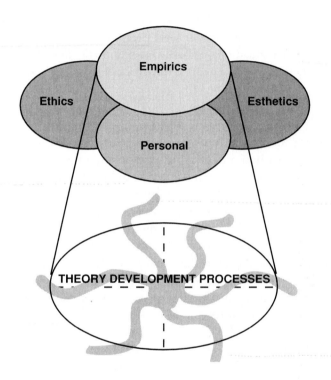

Empiric theory is one expression of the empiric pattern
of knowing. Empiric theory contributes to nursing's
identity, coherence of purpose, and ability to communicate
within nursing and with people in related professions.
Four processes integrate to create empiric
theory. These are influenced by nursing's
heritage, values, and resources that evolve from the past.

In this book, we primarily focus on understanding, developing, and examining the empiric pattern of knowing and the range of theory that ex-presses empiric knowledge. Our discussion of empiric theory draws on generally accepted ideas about scientific theory as well as our own ideas of empiric theory in a human science applied in a practice discipline. Theorizing is often thought of as a cognitive or mental phenomenon, but, in our view, theory is developed by being and acting in the world. We also believe that reasoning, logic, and the experiences of practice must be integrated to express the most useful empiric knowledge.

WHAT IS THEORY?

Defining *theory* can be complex, and ultimately most people accept an arbitrary meaning. Just when a definition seems firm, another idea surfaces that must be integrated into it. Like most terms, theory has many meanings, both within and outside of the profession of nursing. Theory has common, everyday connotations apparent in such phrases as "I have a *theory* about that" or "my *theory* is " These usages imply that theory is an idea or feeling or that it explains something. In this book, we have used a definition that is consistent with these everyday meanings of theory as a collection of ideas or explanatory hunches. But our definition goes beyond this to a characterization of theory as something deliberately designed and created for a specific purpose.

In the broad, generic sense, we have defined *empiric theory* as a systematic abstraction of reality that serves some purpose.

Systematic abstraction suggests both an organized pattern underlying the creation and design of theory, as well as the idea that theory is not reality itself. For example, a mosaic is an art form that represents a type of systematic abstraction. A mosaic does not evolve from haphazardly adding individual tiles to a background. It is created when the designer carefully plans how the tiles should be arranged to form a pattern. The form to be achieved, which exists in the artist's mind, represents an idea or constellation of ideas. Like the mosaic, theory has organization and pattern. The organization of abstract ideas occurs with the use of disciplined, systematic thought and action.

Our broad definition of theory also implies that what is systematized is abstract. It is a representation of reality, not reality itself. The words and other symbols within theory are labels that represent perceptual experiences of objects, properties, or events. For example, the word *book* is a word or label for an object you are presently reading. The word is not the object it represents. To illustrate the difference, close your eyes and conjure an image of a book.

To imagine a book without actually touching or seeing it is a relatively easy task if you have a mental image of what a book is like. You can imagine a book because the word *book* stimulates a mental image or abstraction that represents the object. Theory is made up of words (the label or word *book*) that represent abstractions (mental image of a book) of empiric experiences (object book). The words or symbols that express theory allow those theories to be communicated and understood.

In summary, theory as a systematic abstraction of reality implies an organization of words (or other symbols) that represent perceptual experiences of objects, properties, or events. Because there are many processes by which these abstractions are systematized, theory takes many forms. But the process is always systematic, and the form is always patterned.

Although theory is a systematic abstraction of reality, including nursing reality, it is also purpose-oriented. Just as the processes used in designing theory may vary, the purposes for creating theory will vary. The creative dimensions of empiric theory are description, explanation, and prediction. Description means that abstractions of reality are systematized to account for something—to set forth ideas about what something is. Explanation implies that theory interrelates ideas to account for how something functions. A theory can also predict under what conditions something will occur. These purposes of theory are fundamentally different yet interrelated. To illustrate, think of pain as a central theoretic idea. It is quite a different task to describe pain, to explain how pain occurs, or to predict its occurrence. It is quite possible to predict pain without being able to explain or describe mental and physical processes that determine its manifestations. Descriptions of pain experiences can be extremely useful to nurses and may help nurses account for or predict pain in the absence of explanatory and predictive theory.

WHY DOES NURSING NEED THEORY?

One answer to the question "Why theory in nursing?" is that theory can contribute to a well-founded basis for practice. A common response to questions about the value of theory is to point to past and present problems in nursing that might be solved through theory development or at least partially understood in relation to the presence or absence of theory. For example, many nursing procedures have been ritualistically taught and practiced simply because they have always been done that way. If a theoretic rationale for changing practice is suggested, the alternative can be considered in light of this rationale, and an informed choice can be made about implementing it.

One recurrent myth about theory comes from the tendency to separate the theoretic from the practical, supporting the idea that theory is useless. This myth may be reinforced when broad nursing theories are examined, particularly by a practitioner seeking specific guidelines to assist in practical decisions about nursing care. Some of the practice implications in these theories are not direct or immediately obvious. Formulations that are commonly recognized as nursing theories represent the nursing world as it ought to be or might be, which is different from the nursing world in which practitioners function. As theorists and practitioners work together to understand and develop theories, the nature and form of nursing theory will change, and the theory-practice gap will become increasingly smaller. When a nursing theory is not sufficiently useful, the theory is revised, or the issues about practice that the theory raises are examined. Once practice is viewed in light of theory, the potential becomes more real for theory to be useful in changing practice.

Addressing the question Why is theory useful? can enable both practitioners and theorists to form better relationships between their two worlds. The mere existence of theory provides a sounding board for basic assumptions and values about nurses, nursing, and the ultimate purposes for which nursing practice exists. If a theory seems to lead practice in a direction that is inconsistent with the fundamental caring values of nursing practice, that theory might be rejected, regardless of how well it can be applied in practice.

Theory and professional identity

Theory is important for guiding nursing education, research, and practice and for strengthening the links between nurses in these roles. How theory and identity are linked may be illustrated by considering the general area of family dynamics. Having theoretic knowledge develops an understanding of factors that affects family function. By basing their care on theoretic knowledge about family dynamics, nurses are able to work with families to help create healthy functioning. The effect of theory as a source of professional identity and unity is circular. As theoretic knowledge about family function is refined, nurses develop common understanding about nursing practice with families and base their practice on the theories that are useful. Practice, in turn, influences further development of the theories.

Professional identity that evolves out of theory provides a basis from which nurses can control certain aspects of their practice. Nursing practice has traditionally been controlled by others, and what nurses do is often invisible. Hospital bills, for example, typically do not show nursing costs, leaving the impression that nurses provide no billable services. Theory that guides practice provides a language for talking about the nature of nursing practice and for demonstrating its effectiveness. Once nursing practice is described, it is made visible. When its effectiveness can be shown, it can be deliberately shaped or controlled by those who practice it (Dzurec and Abraham, 1993).

On an individual level, theory can provide self-identity and esteem as a nurse because you will have a firmer base when your ideas are questioned. As you become familiar with the language and processes of theoretic knowledge development, you can begin to think about how assumptions, definitions, and relationships within theories can be challenged. The study and understanding of theory provides a basis on which to take risks, to act deliberately, and to improve practice.

Imagine yourself as a nurse using massage to ease chronic pain for a hospitalized person. A physician discovers that you are using this method of care, which is not medically prescribed. Since this is an unfamiliar approach to the physician, she asks you about it. You explain your reasoning, which is based on theory. You also can provide research evidence of the effectiveness of massage and information about the positive results that this particular person is experiencing. Your explanation leads to an informed discussion about various approaches to caring for people with pain and why your approach seems to be effective for this person. As other practitioners learn of your knowledge in this area, they seek your consultation in caring for people with pain. Your knowledge of pain theory and what is effective in caring for people with pain provides a valuable resource for developing and improving practice.

This incident may be idealistic, but it illustrates the potential of a theoretic foundation for professional identity. Theories, especially those developed and refined in conjunction with practice, provide one avenue for developing both individual and collective identity.

Theory and coherence of purpose

Varying points of view concerning the purpose of nursing are reflected in the following questions:

- Should nurses address prevention of illness?
- Should nurses treat human responses to illness?
- Should educational programs be structured around nursing process? Nursing diagnosis? Patterns of knowing? Critical thinking?
- Should nurses view health and illness as opposites?
- Can ill or diseased people also be healthy?

Coherence of professional purpose is linked to professional identity. Coherence of purpose contributes to a collective identity when nurses agree on the general practice domain. Theory can help resolve significant disagreements among practitioners about what is to be accomplished.

For example, suppose a theory has been developed by and for nurses that directs practice toward health maintenance functions. This theory, in part, defines the parameters of health and is useful in guiding practitioners toward maintaining it. If nurses were to use this theory, health maintenance would emerge as a special expertise of nursing. The emergence of health maintenance as our unique role would be communicated within nursing, with the identity of professional nursing becoming clearer.

Theory facilitates coherence by providing a basis for deliberate choices. Theory directs nursing toward some purpose other than filling in a gap. When nurses agree about professional purposes and develop theory related to those purposes, the public and other practitioners will recognize nursing's expertise in relation to that theoretic arena. The fact that nurses are responsible for certain phenomena will be directly and indirectly communicated to society, and professional identity and coherence of purpose will continue to evolve.

A somewhat simple and imprecise example may help to illustrate the value of theory in developing coherence of purpose. Suppose you wish to drive across the United States from the Pacific coast to the Atlantic coast. Both Maine and Florida are attractive and acceptable destinations, and the people traveling with you have mixed opinions about the merits of each. Your initial decision about where to go is quite separate from the choice of how to get there. Deciding on your destination will influence your decision about the route to take. But, on the other hand, your destination can depend on the options you perceive for getting there. If your group wishes to ride a train and the only train service is to Maine, you might decide on your destination and your route because you want to ride the train. If you decide to get in a car and just drive, with the purpose of experiencing whatever you find across the continent, you are likely to have a good trip, but you will not be able to assure anyone as to where you will be going and when you might arrive.

This example illustrates some of the considerations that nurses might take into account in developing theory. Having a purpose, or a destination, is not essential, but it does help to shape complex decisions when many different people are involved. As coherent purposes for nursing emerge, the means of attaining the goals and the relative merits of journeying one way or another can be carefully considered.

Theory and professional communication

All theory, regardless of type, helps to enhance communication. The study of theory by practicing nurses and students of nursing provides a common foundation of knowledge and thought from which to practice. If knowledge of existing theory within nursing is essential, all students of nursing should be familiar with nursing's theoretic knowledge and understand the basics of theory development.

If theory is to be useful for practice, theorists must be concerned about how theory relates to the practice arena. We believe it is essential to communicate with the world of practice to foster professional communication.

Using the example of pain management, if a theorist were devising a theory to guide the care for people with chronic pain, pain would be an idea (concept) of key importance within the theory. Since the word *pain* represents a complex abstraction, pain alleviation could mean many things. Suppose the theorist intends to develop the theory by using research to test the effectiveness of two or three pain alleviation methods. The theorist and researchers must determine how to empirically represent chronic pain phenomena. Some of the decisions that must be made are (1) how to think about and assess pain, (2) how to relate the pain experience to nursing care modalities, and (3) how to determine pain relief, which in turn would indicate the effectiveness of nursing care.

One choice for assessing pain is to monitor neural response using a skin electrode attached to a laboratory instrument. When assessed this way, pain is seen as an oscilloscope display of frequency and amplitude of action potentials. The effectiveness of the tested nursing care modalities is determined by alterations in the neural response that in turn represent pain.

A second choice for representing pain can be quite different. Rather than an oscilloscope tracing, a score derived from observing body movement and the person's report of the pain experience are used to assess pain. The difference between assessing pain from a neural response and assessing pain from observation of behavior illustrates how the word *pain* can legitimately be assessed in different ways, and either assessment approach is reasonable.

Suppose the research team chooses to assess the effectiveness of two different approaches to nursing care by bringing people to the laboratory and monitoring their neural response using the oscilloscope tracing. When this clinically inaccessible method of assessing pain is chosen, it is difficult to transfer the ideas of the theory into practice. First, variables that operate in the clinical area are not operating in the laboratory setting. Second, the nurses have no way of knowing how neural response patterns relate to the subjective experience of pain. If the research team chooses to use the subjective response scale to represent pain, the theory more readily lends itself to further clinical testing since the pain assessment technique considers the subjective pain response.

When a theory is developed using research, the choices about how to represent ideas (concepts)—in this example, pain—will determine how useful the theory is. A theory that is useful for practice enhances communication between theorists, researchers, and nurses in practice. If theory is to enhance professional communication, it must be developed in a way that maximizes its utility for practice.

Some theories do not initially and immediately address clinical nursing concerns. In fact, theory that is useful for practice can be rooted in research that is quite remote from nursing care environments. Ultimately, however, theory development should arise from some frame of reference that addresses nursing concerns in a way that enhances communication between nurses in practice and those developing the theory.

What kind of theory?

In recent nursing literature, there are discussions about what constitutes *nursing* theory. Should nursing have theories *about* nursing? *For* nursing? Or *in* nursing? Is basic theory important? Is applied theory important? Is broad theory about health care systems important? The answer to these and related questions is—yes! We believe that many types of theory covering many areas are needed in nursing. However, to answer yes to all these questions does little to resolve the difficulty of knowing which choice to make between alternate approaches at any given time. In our opinion, the choice should be guided by an explicit purpose or concern that can be communicated to others and is seen as reasonable or important by others in the discipline.

Theory in nursing contributes to communicating among practitioners, to clarifying the purposes of nursing, and to forming professional identity. Theory is not the only answer, and, as with other professions, there are many personal and political issues that affect its development. The processes and products of theory development build on, but also transcend, the personal and political realities, providing a substantive foundation from which to work.

HOW DOES A DISCIPLINE ACQUIRE THEORY?

There are four processes for creating empiric theory, which are shown as quadrants in Figure 2–1. When all of these processes occur, theory with practical value evolves. Central to each of the processes is a historical core from which curved lines emanate. The wave lines represent current situations and circumstances that have roots in nursing history. The lines separating each quadrant illustrate that each process is different from, but continuous with, other processes. The processes are enclosed by broken lines to symbolize that there is open communication between nursing's theory development processes and similar processes in other professions and disciplines, but that boundaries still exist.

Processes for theory development

Each of four major processes contributes to the development of theory in a practice discipline (see Fig. 2–1). These are (1) creating conceptual meaning,

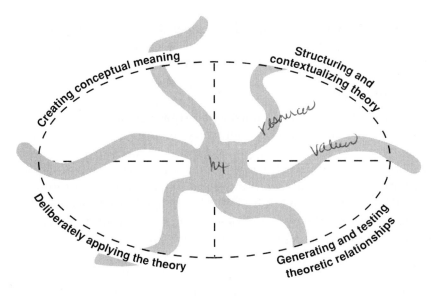

FIGURE 2–1 A process of theory development.

(2) structuring and contextualizing theory, (3) generating and testing theoretic relationships, and (4) deliberately applying the theory.

Creating conceptual meaning. This is a creative process of identifying, examining, and clarifying the mental images that compose the elements, variables, or concepts within theory. This process is used particularly with the major concepts around which a theory is developed.

Structuring and contextualizing theory. This is the process of organizing relationships between and among concepts in a unique, creative, rigorous, and systematic way, consistent with the purposes of the theory. This process also includes identifying the domain, realm, or context of the theory, stating the assumptions on which the theory is based, and providing conceptual definitions of terms that guide decisions about the empiric events to which concepts relate.

Generating and testing theoretic relationships. This process has three subcomponents: (1) empirically grounding emerging relationships, (2) explicating empiric indicators, and (3) validating the relationships through empiric methods.

Deliberately applying the theory. This is the process of using research to evaluate the effectiveness of a theory in achieving the goals of nursing practice. Research can provide evidence of how useful theory is in practice.

A detailed explanation of each of these processes is found in Chapter 5. The remainder of this chapter focuses on other features of the system that symbolize the theory development processes within nursing.

The heritage of history

We have depicted the heritage of nursing's past by a circle in the center of Figure 2–1. Interpretations of history influence the present direction of theory development, and, to a great extent, determine nursing's area of concern. History changes in an accumulative manner; it can be added to but never subtracted from. The historical core has a boundary because, once history is made, it may be reinterpreted but it cannot be changed. Some historical factors influence current theory development more than others. These are shown as wave lines emanating from the historical core.

Wave lines

The wave lines from the inner core extend into each of the theory development processes and are curvilinear to convey the idea of movement. Since history changes over time, its influence on theory changes.

   The wave lines are circumstances that evolve from the past. There are two general types of circumstances—values and resources. Values and resources can be those of the individual, the professional group, or society. All wave lines extend beyond the open boundaries. This represents the idea that historically derived factors that influence the development of theory in nursing reach out to influence other groups with related theoretic concerns. Values and resources that have had a particular influence on nursing theory development are discussed in Chapter 3.

Quadrant lines

The horizontal and vertical lines represent the distinct nature of each process. The lines are not continuous because, even though each process influences and is influenced by the others, the processes are fundamentally different. The outcome of processes within one quadrant cannot be improved by improving the quality of processes within another quadrant. If, for example, the meaning you create for concepts is incomplete, the idea of the concept will not be improved by designing better theoretic relationships. If the meaning you create is incomplete, the relationships generated that depend on those meanings will also be inadequate.

   To illustrate the characteristics of the individuality yet mutual interrelatedness of each of the processes within the system, consider a family of four people. The family members are separate people; if you know one, you do not automatically know the others. Because the family members are mutually interrelated, you can infer characteristics of the group through knowledge of one member. If you know one member's dietary preferences, you have some clues as to what the nutritional patterns of the group might be, but you cannot empirically know until you ask each member or observe each member's behavior.

Each nurse who contributes to theory development will become more experienced and interested in using one or two of the theory development processes. To the extent that every nurse can appreciate the contributions made by all theory development processes, there will be more potential for development of useful theory in nursing.

Boundary lines

The boundary lines in Figure 2–1 that enclose the theory development processes symbolize the idea that the domain of nursing is limited. But, even though the processes are bounded, there is free exchange of theoretic content and processes among different professions and disciplines. Figure 2–2 illustrates how a group with different purposes can overlap theoretically. The labels we have chosen are arbitrary and are not meant to imply the degree or nature of overlap or separateness of the groups. The areas of overlap suggest that professions share areas of interest. The empiric domains of nursing and medicine overlap. Neither can realistically or effectively deal with all aspects of health and illness.

For example, both nursing and medicine are concerned, in part, with human experiences of health and illness. There is a wide range of health and illness experience; nursing and medicine each work with some common and some different aspects of these experiences. The differences are defined by the distinct purposes and aims of each group as a profession. Medicine aims to cure disease; nursing aims to alleviate the suffering that accompanies

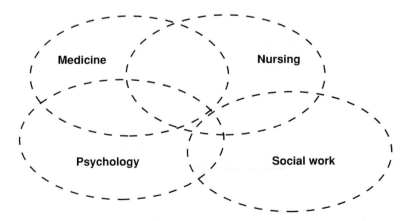

FIGURE 2–2 Overlap of theory development processes among professions.

disease and to promote wellness. Each of these aims is worthy; each concerns the human experience of disease. However, each of these aims is fundamentally different, requiring different types of knowledge and understanding.

USE OF THE PROCESSES FOR THEORY DEVELOPMENT

The processes for theory development are fluid, complex, and diverse. Together, they form a unified whole. Individual nurses, with different talents and aptitudes, can contribute to the process of creating theory. Each individual typically develops skill with respect to one component of the total process. When combined, individual efforts form the whole of the field of inquiry.

Generally, people have an inclination toward one or the other of these processes. If elusive abstract ideas are interesting to you, you may be impatient or bored with research techniques required for testing or applying theory. If you prefer to deal directly with the clinical nursing world, you may be impatient with abstract ideas about practice. Your openness to and your understanding and appreciation of the work of other nurses who use a mode different from yours is a key to creating a cohesive community within nursing. Ideally, individuals with complementary talents and interests will form alliances or channels of communication and will deliberately assist one another. Literature that reflects diverse interests will facilitate understanding and cooperation among nurses. Researchers can benefit from philosophic and analytic work that focuses on the meanings of concepts. Theorists can use research reports as evidence that theories are empirically meaningful. Practitioners can use theory to create new approaches in practice. Each of the processes, occurring in synchrony, can provide unity of purpose for nursing.

work together

CONCLUSION

Empiric theory, the focus for this book, is one expression of empirics. Empiric theory contributes to the identity and coherence of purpose of nursing and to the ability to communicate within nursing and with people in related professions. There are four major processes that are used to develop empiric theory. These processes are creating conceptual meaning, structuring and contextualizing theory, generating and testing theoretic relationships, and deliberately applying the theory. The processes are influenced by nursing historical heritage and the values and resources that evolve from the past.

REFERENCES

Dzurec LC and Abraham IL: The nature of inquiry: linking quantitative and qualitative research, *Adv Nurs Sci 16(1): 73–79, 1993.*

3

Emergence of nursing theory

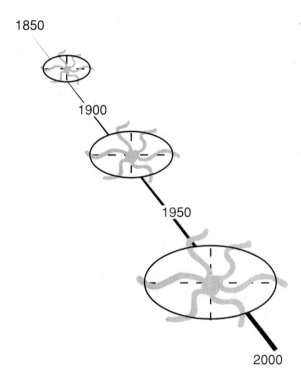

1850

1900

1950

2000

The values and resources influencing theory development
are rooted in history. As early theorists developed a sense
of community and scholarship, they influenced more
recent theoretic developments. A perspective of history
makes it possible to refine understanding of what theory is.

Current issues in nursing can be directly traced to the past and will continue to shape the future. Theory development draws directly on history and the circumstances that evolve from it. This chapter examines the history of nursing and the historically significant values and resources that affect theory development within the profession.

HISTORY OF THEORY DEVELOPMENT

Early in the development of nursing as a profession, leaders in nursing theorized about the nature of nursing practice, the principles on which practice is based, and the proper goals and functions of nursing in society. Early conceptualizations of nursing emphasized the art of nursing. By the 1950s, nurses began to develop nursing science. Professional development and the development of nursing theory have a long and important history (Ashley, 1976).

Nightingale (1969, p. 3), in establishing the discipline of nursing, spoke with firm conviction about the nature of nursing as a profession distinct from medicine. Nightingale conceived of nursing as a profession that could provide an avenue for women to make a meaningful contribution to society.

In the mid-1800s, women cared for the English sick as daughters, wives, mothers, or maids. This socially prescribed role influenced Nightingale's conviction that nursing should be a profession for women, but this cultural tradition was secondary to her philosophy. Her primary concern was the more pervasive plight of Victorian women. Women in her era were either poverty-stricken and forced to work at menial labor for long hours, or they were idle ornaments in the households of wealthy husbands or fathers. In either case, there was no avenue in which women could use their "intellect, passion, and moral activity" to benefit society (Nightingale, 1980).

Nightingale spent the first decade of her adult life tormented by a desire to use her productive capacities in a way that would benefit society. She defied the wishes of her family and obtained formal training as a nurse and subsequently agreed to serve in the Crimean War (Nightingale, 1980; Tooley, 1905; Woodham-Smith, 1983). After her service in the war, Nightingale wrote *Notes on Nursing*, in which she set forth the basic premises on which nursing practice was to be based and articulated the proper functions of nursing. In her view, nursing functions included making astute observations of the sick and their environment, recording observations, and developing knowledge about the factors that promote the reparative process (Nightingale, 1969).

Firmly committed to the idea that nursing's responsibilities were distinct from those of medicine, Nightingale maintained that the knowledge developed and used by nursing must be distinct from medical knowledge. She insisted that women who were trained nurses control and staff early nursing schools, and manage and control nursing practice in homes and hospitals. Nightingale influenced the establishment of schools of nursing in England and the United States. The first Nightingale schools were autonomous in their administration, and nurses held decision-making authority over nursing practice in institutions where students learned. Student learning in these schools emphasized the powers of observation, the necessity of recording observations, and the potential for organizing nursing knowledge gained through observation and recording. In addition, Nightingale held strong beliefs about the values that should be cultivated in nursing, and these values were reflected in the educational programs of early schools (Barnard and Neal, 1977; Dennis and Prescott, 1985).

After the Nightingale era, many forces in society emerged in opposition to Nightingale's model. In the United States, the medical care system developed as a capitalist, for-profit business. This system provided the context for rapid technologic development and a complex industrial system to support medical interventions. Early in the 1900s, when the medical care system was taking shape as a science and as a political body, physicians and hospital administrators saw nurses as a source of inexpensive or free labor who could further their economic goals. Many women who entered nursing and who provided free student labor for hospitals were working-class women with limited opportunities for education. Nurses were exploited both as students and as trained, experienced workers and were viewed as submissive, obedient, and humble women who ideally fulfilled their responsibilities to physicians without question. Nurses' positive desire to help people in need, coupled with a relative lack of educational preparation and social or political power, led to an extended period in history when nursing was practiced primarily under the control and direction of medicine (Lovell, 1980).

Despite strong leaders who followed the Nightingale tradition and viewed nursing knowledge as unique, nursing's knowledge has not always been regarded as distinct from medicine. During the early 1900s, most of the Nightingale-modeled schools in the United States were brought under the control of hospitals, and nursing education and practice were transferred from the profession to the control of hospital administrators and physicians (Ashley, 1976). Consistent with the social history of women, nursing was viewed increasingly as a role supporting and supplementing medicine (Hughes, 1980; Lovell, 1980). Education for women and nurses was discouraged and limited. Women who were nurses were expected to follow orders and serve the needs and interests of physicians providing care (Melosh, 1982; Reverby, 1987). Economic independence for women was not possible until the mid-l900s. Even though a woman earned an income, she was not able to have a bank account, own property, or conduct financial transactions in her own name. Normal schools were established for the training of teachers, and nursing schools were available for training nurses, but to obtain long-term security, women were required to conform to the role of wife or daughter.

Throughout the early part of the twentieth century, nursing practice was based on rules, principles, and traditions that were passed along through limited apprenticeship forms of education. Further education was not available; thus, much of what evolved as nursing knowledge was wisdom that came from years of experience. Principles for practice were sometimes derived from scientific knowledge. Many principles were generalizations from the theories of other disciplines, such as Ohm's law related to pressure, resistance, and flow. Other principles came from generally accepted facts, such as the fact that microbes could be transferred by object-to-object contact or by droplets in the air. Certain traditions of practice were thought to be sound but were never examined. For example, knowledge of the germ theory of disease and related propositions concerning the transmission of disease led to aseptic procedures in handling equipment, isolating individuals who were thought to be contagious, and hand-washing techniques. These approaches became traditions of practice because they were thought to be effective or sound.

Tradition as a basis for nursing practice was perpetuated by the nature of apprenticeship education in nursing (Ashley, 1976). Student nurses were presumed to learn at random through long hours of experience, with limited exposure to lectures or books, and to accept without question the prescriptions of practical techniques. The novice nurse acquired knowledge of what was right and wrong in practice by observing more experienced practitioners and by memorizing facts about the performance of nursing tasks. Nursing was viewed primarily as a nurturing and technical art requiring apprenticeship learning and innate personality traits congruous with the art (Ashley, 1976; Hughes, 1980).

Despite social impediments to the development of nursing knowledge, nursing philosophy and ideology remained committed to the idea that nursing requires a distinct body of knowledge for practice (Abdellah, 1969; Hall, 1964; Henderson, 1964, 1966; Rogers, 1970). This commitment grew from the consistently observed fact that, although the goals of nursing and medicine were similar and related, the central goals and functions of nursing required knowledge not provided by medicine or by any other single discipline outside of nursing.

Despite the social circumstances that limited nursing education, nursing leaders sustained ideals that reflected Nightingale's model of education and practice. Because most nursing service was provided as free labor by students in hospitals, graduate nurses functioned as independent practitioners engaged by families to assist in the care of the sick in homes and in hospitals. Nurse leaders became active in confronting a wide range of social and health issues of the time, including temperance, freedom for slaves, suffrage for blacks and women, and control of venereal disease.

There is substantial evidence that graduate nurses in the early part of the twentieth century contributed substantively to improving health conditions in hospitals, homes, and communities. They developed health knowledge and were politically active in finding ways to distribute this knowledge to people who needed it (Wheeler, 1985).

Consistently throughout the twentieth century, nursing leaders in the United States have worked together nationally and internationally in strong connecting networks calling for social and political reforms to restore the control of nursing practice to nurses. Margaret Sanger, Lillian Wald, and Lavinia Dock are three nurses who led this effort early in the century. These nurses were challenged by specific needs of society and independently set about to develop their practice on the basis of what they saw as a need in health care. They observed the circumstances of people in their communities, identified a health-related need, and organized nurses to meet the needs. They recorded their observations and the conclusions they drew from these observations. Sanger, for example, developed knowledge about reproduction and birth control. She fought against great odds to distribute birth control information to women who were desperate to obtain it and established a foundation for family planning programs that remains viable today (Sanger, 1971).

Wald became concerned about child care and family health in the context of extremely poor conditions of sanitation in the crowded immigrant tenements of New York City. She established the Henry Street Settlement in New York City from which she developed concepts of community health nursing and social welfare programs. She developed stations from which safe milk was distributed to families with young children and centers for educating mothers in the care of their families (Silverstein, 1985; Wald, 1971).

Dock was an ardent suffragist and pacifist who worked with Wald at the Henry Street Settlement. While at Henry Street, she campaigned actively for changes in labor laws that would benefit women and children. She devoted twenty years of her life to gain enfranchisement for women in the United States. Dock reasoned that if women could vote, the oppressive laws that affected them would be changed (Christy, 1969).

Lydia Hall is a more recent example of a nurse who constructed specific philosophic ideas about how nursing should be practiced, and she implemented this philosophy in practice. She established Loeb Center at Montefiore Hospital in New York City, a nursing center where nursing maintains control over the care provided and where people and their families have primary decision-making power over the kind of care that they receive (Hall, 1963).

Like theorists of today, these early nursing leaders developed and used knowledge as one means to bring about improvements in health care and nursing practice. They were convinced that nurses can and should control nursing practice, based on a strong knowledge base. They advocated that nursing practice include making detailed observations, recording these observations, organizing the knowledge that came from their observations, and establishing guiding values and philosophies for practice.

Although many valuable traditions of nursing practice remain, the ideas of nursing as a science that began to take hold in the 1960s produced a significant change. Gradually, nursing shifted from a perspective that emphasized technical competence, duty, and virtue to a questioning perspective that focuses more on what is effective nursing practice (Hardy, 1978).

The shift toward science as the basis for developing nursing knowledge was influenced by the involvement of nursing in the two world wars of the 1900s. The wars created social circumstances that brought about substantial shifts in roles for women and nurses. During wars, women were relatively free to manage their responsibilities in accord with their own priorities and preferences. Many women entered the skilled or unskilled labor force during the years when men were away in battle. Women who were nurses were needed to support the war effort by providing care for the sick and wounded. War-related programs were instituted by the U.S. government to make nursing preparation available to women who agreed to serve in the war (Kalisch and Kalisch, 1978; Kelly, 1992).

Partly because of the greater demand for skilled nurses to serve the war effort, by the decade of World War II, women had begun to enter institutions of higher learning in greater numbers. Nursing leaders conceived of nursing education as being properly placed within colleges and universities. Early efforts to develop nursing research began in the context of the military, which provided support for nursing research.

After the end of World War II, many educational programs were established within institutions of higher learning rather than in hospitals, and graduate programs for nurses began to appear. Academic institutions required faculty to hold advanced degrees and encouraged them to meet the standards of higher education with regard to service to community, teaching, research, and scholarship. Once nurses gained skills in the methods of science, nursing theories and other types of theoretic writings appeared.

In 1950, *Nursing Research*, the first nursing research journal, was established. Books on research methods and explicit theories of nursing began to appear. Early research reports are less sophisticated in method when compared to those of today, but these writings quickly changed and began to reflect qualities of serious scholarship and investigative skill. Various schools of thought emerged about the nature of nursing practice, providing a fresh flow of ideas that could be examined by members of the profession. These writings provided a stimulus for early efforts in developing theory.

By the 1960s, doctoral programs in nursing were being established. With this development, committees of nurses began to formally consider the development of nursing knowledge. Nurse scholars began to debate ideas, points of view, and methods in the light of nursing's traditions (Hardy, 1978; Leininger, 1976). These debates are reflected in the literature of the late 1960s and early 1970s (Dickoff and James, 1971; Dickoff, James, and Wiedenbach, 1968; Ellis, 1971; Folta, 1971; Walker 1971, 1972; Wooldridge, 1971). Fundamental differences in viewpoints about nursing science provided nurse scholars the opportunity to learn, sharpen critical-thinking skills, and acquire knowledge about the processes of science.

By the end of the 1970s, the number of doctorally prepared nurses in the United States had grown to nearly 2,000. Approximately twenty doctoral programs in nursing had been established, and masters programs were maturing in academic stature and quality. Masters programs were focused on preparing advanced practitioners in nursing rather than on preparing educators and administrators.

TRENDS IN THEORY DEVELOPMENT

Throughout the second half of the twentieth century, there were four major trends that contributed to evolving directions in developing nursing knowledge. These trends were (1) the development of conceptual models and philosophies of practice, (2) the application of theories borrowed from other disciplines, (3) the development of theories broadly defining the discipline, and (4) the development of midrange theory linked to practice.

Conceptual models and philosophies of practice

First, nurses began to reconsider the nature of nursing and the purposes for which nursing exists. Nurses began to question the ideas that were taken for granted in nursing and the traditional basis on which nursing was practiced. They wrote and published their ideas about nursing and the type of knowledge, skills, and background needed for practice. Although many of the writings of the 1960s and 1970s were not intended as theories in a formal sense, they are significant contributions to the development of theoretic thinking in nursing. Many of these theoretic works have been used as a basis for curricula, and some have been applied in practice.

Many early nursing conceptual models and philosophies include a description of the nursing process. This process, which is similar to both the problem-solving and the research processes, is a framework for viewing nursing as a deliberate, reflective, critical, and self-correcting system. The nursing process replaced the rule- and principle-oriented approaches that were grounded in a concept of the nurse as a physician extender. Rules and principles were followed as the nurse performed procedures and gave medications to treat disease. A rule-oriented approach did not encourage reflective problem solving. The shift to the nursing process as a way to approach care encouraged nurses to cultivate basic inquiry skills. Nursing diagnosis, which evolved from the nursing process and began to move nursing away from dependence on a medical model, was one means for organizing the domain of nursing practice. The early literature concerning nursing diagnosis included practical and theoretic ideas about developing a taxonomy of nursing diagnoses and testing their validity.

Conceptual models for nursing education and practice proliferated in the 1960s and 1970s. Philosophies of nursing science and nursing practice developed, with growing emphasis on esthetic, ethical, and personal components of nursing knowledge. As these ideas began to be used in practice settings, the relationships between nursing models and nursing practice have become clearer. Practicing nurses found a new sense of purpose and direction consistent with the basic values of nursing and a sense of the increasing effectiveness achieved through use of systematic and thoughtful forms of nursing practice. The ideas of Sister Callista Roy, Dorothea Orem, Betty Neuman, and Imogene King are examples of theoretic ideas that have been applied in practice.

The application of theories borrowed from other disciplines

As the educational preparation of nurses expanded, theories that had been developed in other disciplines were recognized as important for nursing. Problems in nursing practice for which there had seemed no readily available solution began to be viewed as resolvable if theories from other disciplines were applied. For example, nurses recognized that young children needed the continuing love and support of their parents and families during hospitalization. The strict rules of hospitals that severely restricted visitation interrupted these primary family ties. As psychological theories of attachment and separation developed, nurses found an explanation for the problems experienced by hospitalized children and were able to change visitation practices to provide sustained contact between parents and children.

Although theories from other disciplines have been useful in some instances, nurses have also exercised caution in arbitrarily applying these theories. In some instances, the theories of other disciplines do not take into consideration significant factors that influence a nursing situation. For example, some theories of learning applicable to classroom learning do not adequately reflect the process of learning when an individual is faced with the stress of an illness. Although borrowed theories may be useful, their usefulness cannot be assumed until they are examined from the perspective of nursing in nursing situations (Whall, 1980).

The development of theory broadly defining the discipline

The early formal movement to develop theory originating from nursing was influenced by the writings of Dickoff and James and their colleagues. They described one view of how theory can be developed and the nature of theory for a practice discipline (Dickoff and James, 1968; Dickoff, James, and Wiedenbach, 1968). Their approaches were discussed in the literature and at conferences, reflecting a growing commitment of nurses to develop nursing theory, or theory derived directly from practice, and defining what nursing practice should consist of.

Other approaches to developing theory broadly defining practice combined direct observations of practice, insights derived from existing theories and other literature sources, and insights derived from explicit philosophic perspectives about nursing and the nature of health and human experience. Nursing theories developed in the 1960s and 1970s broadly defined nursing and named the phenomena central to nursing's domain of concern. These theories described how nursing functions to achieve a socially relevant purpose and described the explanations of the contextual variables important to the practice of nursing. There is a philosophic component in early nursing theories that reflects assumptions and values on which nursing rests. At the same time, early theories are characterized by a relatively functional view of nursing and health that defines what nursing is, describes the social purposes nursing serves, and describes how nurses function to realize these purposes, and defined the parameters and variables influencing illness and health processes.

For example, the theories of Sister Callista Roy, Dorothea Orem, Virginia Henderson, and Hildegard Peplau focus on descriptions of illness and health, describing what nurses do to assist the person to move toward health. These theories present explanations of how nursing actions function to enhance health and well-being. The functions described are theoretic in nature, in that they are conceptualized at a relatively abstract level. Nursing is viewed as types of roles and functions, not as concrete nursing procedures. These abstract ideas about nursing functions are woven into explanations of relationships between the function and the theorist's idea of a desired nursing outcome related to health and well-being.

In the later 1970s and 1980s, there is a noticeable qualitative shift in theories developed for the purpose of broadly defining nursing. Rather than reflect a functional perspective of the role of nursing in society, the later theories tend to move to qualitative dimensions that characterize nursing's role not as what nurses do, but as the essence of what nursing is. This shift offers potential for moving nursing from a context-dependent reactive position to a context-independent proactive stance.

For example, both Jean Watson and Patricia Benner have developed theories of nursing that ground the essence of nursing in caring. Each of these theorists use theoretical reasoning that is derived from a deliberate philosophic stance and from experience of the practice of nursing in many different contexts. The themes or patterns that characterize the essence of caring theory are those reflected in the actions, thoughts, values, and priorities of the practicing nurse.

The development of midrange practice-linked theory

During the 1980s, Meleis (1987) brought into a clear focus the need for nurses to develop substantive theory that provides a meaningful foundation for the development of nursing practice in relation to specific phenomena. In accord with the observation of many practicing nurses, Meleis acknowledged the value of broad-scope theories in defining general parameters on which nursing function is based but noted that theory of a different type was required to give more specific guidance for nursing practice. She called for substance in theory, which focuses on concepts grounded in a practice context.Theory of this type coincides with research questions directly linked to important practice problems. It avoids a focus on methodology and shifts the focus to understanding phenomena. This understanding can inform practice and lead to new practice approaches by exploring various factors that influence the outcomes desired in nursing practice.

Midrange theory tends to cluster around a concept of interest, such as social support, pain, grief, fatigue, or life transitions. Several nurse researcher/scholars may work in concert with practitioner/scholars to develop theory related to a substantive area of concern. Each theorist's perspective contributes to developing research, theory, and practice in the substantive area.

MAJOR VIEWS EXPRESSED IN NURSING THEORY

From these developments in the history of nursing, philosophic foundations evolved that are now common elements in nursing theories and models. They include ideas about the nature of nursing, the nature of the person, society and environment, and health (Fawcett, 1978; Yura and Torres, 1975). The manner in which each of these ideas has been developed characterizes the nature of nursing as a distinct discipline and provides direction for the future development of nursing knowledge.

Nature of nursing

In nursing theory, nursing is generally represented as a helping process with a primary focus on interpersonal interactions between a nurse and another individual. This general idea does not clearly distinguish nursing from other helping disciplines, but it provides an important focus for deciding what kind of knowledge is needed in nursing practice. The interpersonal nature of nursing practice distinguishes nursing from medicine, in that medicine focuses on surgical and pharmacological interventions with interpersonal interactions secondary to these interventions. For nursing, interpersonal interactions are primary; technical and medical interventions support the primary interpersonal interactions.

Ideas in theoretic writings related to the nature of nursing are significant indicators of the esthetic component of nursing knowledge. For example, Ernestine Wiedenbach (1964) views nursing action taken in response to a person's need as a visible expression of the art of nursing. Hildegard Peplau (1952), Joyce Travelbee (1966, 1971), Josephine Paterson and Loretta Zderad (1976), Rosemarie Parse (1987), Jean Watson (1985), and Patricia Benner (1984) have provided additional important contributions to conceptualizing the art of nursing.

Although different nurse authors present conceptualizations of the nature of nursing that are consistent with the idea of interpersonal interactions as a primary focus, there are important differences in their definitions and conceptualizations. For some authors, the direction of the interaction and the specific actions that are taken in achieving the goals of the interaction are largely defined by the person with whom the nurse interacts. The nurse's role in the interaction is primarily one of facilitating. When this view of the nature of nursing is incorporated into a theory or model, nursing is viewed as enabling the will and behavior of the person receiving care.

Other theories present a view of the interpersonal process as one that is either shared or initiated by the nurse. In this view, nursing processes and actions rest primarily on the nurse's initiative, knowledge, and approaches. The theoretic ideas that emerge from this view focus on nursing actions to reach the goal of the interaction.

Each of these perspectives is consistent with the practice of nursing in that nurses encounter some situations in which the client primarily directs the interaction and others in which the nurse is the initiator. Some nursing theories account for this diversity. The common thread that is significant is the view of the primacy of human interaction in creating human health and wholeness. Table 3–1 describes the concept of nursing as reflected in the work of several nurse theorists.

Table 3–1 Theoretic ideas about nursing

Author	Concepts of nursing
Hildegard Peplau (1952)	Nursing is a significant therapeutic interpersonal process. The interpersonal process is a maturing force and educative instrument for both the nurse and the client. Self-knowledge in the context of the interpersonal interaction is essential to understanding the client and reaching resolution of the problem. There are four sequential phases of the interpersonal process: (1) orientation, (2) identification, (3) exploitation, and (4) resolution.
Ida Jean Orlando (1961)	Nursing is a process of interaction with an ill individual to meet an immediate need. The nursing situation consists of (1) the person's behavior, (2) the nurse's reaction, and (3) nursing action appropriate to the person's need. The nurse is accountable to the individual receiving care.
Ernestine Wiedenbach (1964)	There are three components of nursing: (1) identification of a person's need for help, (2) ministration of the help needed, and (3) validation that the help provided was indeed helpful. The nursing process begins with an activating situation that arouses the nurse's consciousness. Clinical nursing has four components—philosophy, purpose, practice, and art.
Myra Levine (1967)	Nursing care is both supportive and therapeutic. Supportive interventions are designed to maintain a state of wholeness as consistently as possible with failing adaptation. Therapeutic interventions are designed to promote adaptation that contributes to health and restoration of health. All nursing actions are based on conservation of energy, structural integrity, personal integrity, and social integrity.
Jean Watson (1985)	Nursing is a human science and an art that is based on the moral ideal and value of caring. There are 10 carative factors that constitute the knowledge and practice of human care nursing. The context of nursing is humanitarian and metaphysical; the goal of nursing is to gain a higher degree of harmony in mind, body, and soul, which leads to self-knowledge, self-reverence, self-healing, and self-care.

The person

All nursing theories and models include ideas about the nature of human beings. The most consistent philosophic component of the idea of the person is the dimension of wholeness, or holism. The nature of holism as a concept is difficult to address from the perspective of traditional Western philosophies based on the idea of reductionism. In the reductionist view of holism, the whole is equal to the sum of the parts; when interrelationships among parts are understood, generalizations can be made about the whole (Newman, 1979). Western culture is based on this view, in that nurses, like others in this culture, have learned to think about parts of lives, parts of bodies, and parts of human experiences.

In a pure sense, holism means that the whole is greater than the sum of the parts and that the whole cannot be reduced to parts without losing something in the process. Some nursing theorists view the individual as a system of biologic, sociologic, and psychologic parts. This view is not consistent with holism in its purest sense, but there is still a strong commitment to the idea that all components of the individual need to be considered (Flaskerud and Halloran, 1980). Martha Rogers, Margaret Newman, Joyce Travelbee, and Patricia Benner are examples of nurse scholars whose work reflects a view that the individual is different from and greater than the sum of the parts. Table 3–2 describes the concept of person as reflected in the work of several nurse theorists.

Society and environment

The concept of society and environment is consistently viewed as central to the discipline of nursing. These concepts are not addressed as fully in some writings as in others. Several nursing theories deal with the concept of society, or culture, and view it as a critical interacting force shaping the individual (Table 3–3). The environment was central for Nightingale in her concepts of nursing. Nightingale believed that the primary focus for nursing was to alter the physical environment to place the human body in the best possible condition for the reparative processes of nature to occur. Several early contemporary nurse authors gave less emphasis to environment per se or viewed it as encompassing the notion of society, sometimes using the word society to include environment. However, the concept of environment has reemerged as a significant one, particularly in the work of Martha Rogers and theorists who build on her ideas.

Health

The concept of health is usually identified as the goal of nursing. Nightingale stated "the same laws of health or of nursing, for in reality they are the same, obtain among the well as among the sick" (Nightingale, 1969, p. 9). Contemporary nursing theories are remarkably congruous with this early conceptualization. Some theories and models are based on a conceptualization of

Table 3–2 Theoretic ideas about the person

Author	Concepts of person
Joyce Travelbee (1966)	A single human being, family, or community whose illness experience has unique meaning
Virginia Henderson (1966)	Mind and body are inseparable. No two individuals are alike; each is unique. The individual's basic needs are reflected in 14 components of basic nursing care.
Martha Rogers (1970)	Unitary human being is viewed as an energy field, the boundaries of which extend beyond the discernible mass of the human body. There are five unifying assumptions about the life process: (1) unified wholeness, (2) openness, (3) unidirectionality, (4) pattern and organization, and (5) sentience.
Dorothea Orem (1971)	The individual is an integrated whole composed of an internal physical, psychologic, and social nature with varying degrees of self-care ability.
Imogene King (1971)	Individuals are viewed as (1) reacting beings, (2) time-oriented beings, and (3) social beings, with the ability to perceive, think, feel, choose, set goals, and make decisions.
Patricia Benner and Judith Wrubel (1989)	The person is a self-interpreting being engaged in the world. Engagement is possible because of the human capacities of embodied intelligence, culturally acquired meanings, concern, and direct involvement in or grasp of a situation.

a health-illness continuum, and nursing's purpose is to assist the ill client to achieve the highest degree of health possible. Other nurse authors view the concept of health as something more than, or different from, the absence of disease. It exists independently from illness or disease. In these views, health is a dynamic process that changes with time and varies according to life circumstances. Some authors view the health process as interdependent with circumstances of the environment, whereas others view the health process as something that originates with the individual (Smith, 1983).

In an attempt to deal more specifically with ideas related to health, several nurse authors avoid using the terms *health* and *illness*. An example is Levine's (1967) use of the term *conserving holism*. This concept directs nurses to focus on the totality of a person's situation rather than on the typical parameters that have come to be commonly known as health. Table 3–4 identifies

Table 3–3 Theoretic ideas about society and environment

Author	Concepts of society/environment
Florence Nightingale (1860)	Environment is the central concept. It is viewed as all external conditions and influences affecting life and the development of the organism. The major emphasis is on warmth, effluvia (odors), noise, and light.
Joyce Travelbee (1966)	Environment is the context in which human-to-human relatedness or rapport is established.
Myra Levine (1967)	Society is viewed as the total environment of the individual, including family, significant others, and the nurse.
Sister Callista Roy (1976)	Environment constantly interacts with the individual and determines, in part, adaptation level. Stimuli originate in the environment.
Margaret Newman (1986)	Environment and person form a unitary pattern that is reflected in movement-space-time patterns of consciousness. Environment encompasses the total situation and is one with the person; environment includes the universe.

Table 3–4   Theoretic ideas about health

Author	Terms related to health
Lydia Hall (1966)	Self-actualization, self-love
Virginia Henderson (1966)	Independent function
Myra Levine (1967)	Maintaining holism/conservation
Dorothea Orem (1971)	Self-care agency
Josephine Paterson and Loretta Zderad (1976)	Authentic awareness
Sister Callista Roy (1976)	Continual adaptation
Margaret Newman (1986)	Expanding consciousness

some of the terms that nurses have used in constructing their theoretic ideas about health. These terms suggest ideas that more specifically reflect nursing's concerns and de-emphasize the focus on disease or illness.

THE DISCIPLINE OF NURSING: PHILOSOPHY OF DEVELOPMENT OF NURSING KNOWLEDGE

A discipline is characterized by collective knowledge development among persons within a common interest area. One trait that distinguishes a discipline from other social groups is that a disciplinary group has as its purpose developing theory and knowledge. Groups of people, such as bridge clubs or church congregations, who have common interests are social groups. People in these groups sometimes take on projects that involve improving their knowledge and skill related to specific interests, but their primary purpose for forming the group is not to develop new knowledge. An occupational group is formed by individuals who share certain job-related skills and knowledge. Hairdressers, office workers, or real estate agents constitute occupational groups. People in these groups engage in learning activities to acquire and update skills and understandings.

Groups whose purpose is to produce new theory and knowledge within an area of inquiry are known as disciplines. Professions, such as social work, nursing, or medicine, are composed of people who practice and develop new knowledge to be used in their practice. Scholars who create knowledge also select and create knowledge-development methods that are suited to the requirements of the practice and propose the standards by which the knowledge of the discipline is judged to be worthwhile (Donaldson and Crowley, 1978). Early and contemporary nursing theorists and philosophers provide a significant foundation from which nursing continues to evolve as a discipline. Their writings form the characteristics of nursing's knowledge. Within this common frame of reference, there is a great deal of room for diversity of views, which creates new and more useful ideas as the practice of nursing changes.

The nature of key nursing concepts and holism

A major philosophic dilemma in the development of new knowledge in any field is how to determine what kinds of knowledge and approaches to developing knowledge are most valuable. This dilemma is evident when the nature of primary concepts within the discipline of nursing is considered. A key example is the concept that nursing has of the individual as a holistic being. The methods of science, as well as the criteria by which the methods are judged as being adequate, have traditionally been based on objective observation of discrete elements, deliberately isolated from the whole.

The concept of a holistic _person_ means that nothing is reduced to discrete elements or isolated from its context (Francis, 1980; Kramer, 1990; Newman, 1979; Winstead-Fry, 1980) . The concepts of _health_ that have emerged in nursing imply a movement toward wholeness. The concept that the totality of the _environment_ and the place of the person in _society_ contributes to wholeness indicates that nursing must view the individual and the environment as an integral whole.

Moccia (1988) observed that choosing methods for developing nursing knowledge is not based solely on technical considerations. Rather, the choices we make in method represent significant philosophic issues that concern the nature of what it means to be human. From this perspective, nursing cannot patch traditional scientific methods together with newer methods of inquiry to achieve methods that are consistent with a view of human wholeness. She states:

> The dilemma that has finally been uncovered by the methods debate is whether science and professionalism are designed and/or able to serve humanity or whether they will instead serve those with the power to define and control what is meant by science and professionalism.... If the goal of [nursing] practice is to assist people in developing potential that is uniquely theirs, then research is needed that will give researchers and providers information to enhance the depth and complexity of their understanding of individual instances. The choice is how to become more fully engaged in the lives of those who are to receive nursing care rather than more completely distanced from their daily activities (Moccia, 1988, p. 7).

Several nurse scholars have proposed methods or approaches to the development of nursing knowledge that are consistent with the philosophic meanings of the concept of holism. Criticisms of the methods and approaches of traditional science that appeared in nursing literature have clarified the essential problems, making way for proposals for alternative methods (Benner, 1985; Bramwell, 1984; Engel, 1984; Jacobs, 1986; Moccia, 1985; Stevens, 1989).

Several innovative methods have been developed within the philosophic perspective of holism. Margaret Newman (1979) proposed that a holistic approach requires identifying patterns that reflect the whole. Patricia Benner and Judith Wrubel (1989) proposed a phenomenologic/hermeneutic method of inquiry that rests on the meaning of experience as primary to all else, grounding the view of the person within that total context and the meanings of that context.

The methods of theory development that we propose integrate the personal, esthetic, ethical, and empiric patterns of knowing and reflect how we address the inclusion of methods that are congruous with holism. Integration of different patterns of knowing enables choices that are congruous with the tenets of holism.

THE CONTEXTS OF THEORY DEVELOPMENT

Nursing history creates specific circumstances and contexts that influence the development of theory. These include professional, individual, and societal values and resources. Table 3–5 lists values and resources that continue to influence the development of theory in nursing.

Table 3–5 Values and resources that influence theory development

Wave lines	Examples of specific factors
	VALUES
Individual	Commitment to the discipline
	Philosophy of nursing
	Motives
	World view or philosophy
	Priorities for action
Professionl	Commitment to development of knowledge
	Code of ethics
	Standards for practice
	Standards for human research participants
	Willingness to challenge social traditions
	Priorities for allocating the resources of the professional group
Societal	Cultural mores
	Ethical codes
	Priorities for allocating resources
	RESOURCES
Individual	Cognitive style
	Intellectual ability
	Personality
	Lifestyle and setting
	Educational background
	Life experience
	Economic power
Professional	Educational requirements for members
	Body of literature and communication style
	Methodologies and instrumentation
	Practice traditions
	Group profile in relation to education, economic power, political influence
Societal	Settings for practice, education, and research
	Funding for the discipline's activities
	Material requirements

Values

Individual values include an individual's commitment, motives, personal philosophy, beliefs, and priorities. Professional values are beliefs and ideologies that are generally held in common by members of the profession and are used to guide professional action. They are expressed in formal statements issued by professional groups in the form of codes, standards of practice, and ethical theory and are also reflected in repeated themes that occur in the literature and in the collective actions taken by professional organizations.

Societal values are ideologies expressed through societal choices, sanctions, and mores during a given period in history. When individual, professional, and societal values are basically congruous, there is relative stability, and new insights tend to build on what is already established as knowledge in the discipline. When individual, professional, or societal values conflict with one another, the potential exists for creating fundamental change in knowledge and in practice.

Resources

Resources can also be viewed as individual, professional, and societal. Individual resources include the natural and acquired talents shared among members of the discipline, including cognitive style, intellectual abilities, life circumstances, and educational preparation. The collective membership of the discipline forms the professional resources that support ongoing theory development. Examples of professional resources include a growing body of literature and practice traditions, the ability to communicate these among members of the profession, the educational attainments of members of the profession and the nature of that education, and methodologies and instrumentation available for theory development.

Societal resources are those circumstances, materials, space, and funds acquired by the profession from the society at large. Acquisition of societal resources depends on features of the society and the profession. For example, political influence is required to obtain funds, materials, and space to carry out the activities of the discipline. If the political system of society reflects priorities other than those that concern nursing, societal resources are less available to nursing than to other groups that reflect those priorities.

The problem of allocating resources illustrates the circular relationship between resources and values. Politics involves value decisions about who does and does not deserve the resources of society. If, as the course of history shows, women scientists are consistently provided limited or no resources of society, the ability of women to influence value decisions is lessened. Nursing

is a group comprised mostly of women (a professional resource) within a societal context that devalues women as scientists. This influences the profession's ability to exert influence on society at large and gain access to
resources. The contemporary women's movement has created a stimulus for
recognizing societal restrictions on nursing as a sex-segregated occupation
and the effects of systematic oppression of nurses and nursing (Greenleaf,
1980; Roberts, 1983). Feminist theory, which shares many of the traits of nursing theory, provides a perspective for changing social values and shifting social resources. Feminism places on society an urgent demand for a values
transformation that is consistent with nursing's vision of health, the health
care system, and nursing (Chinn and Wheeler, 1985). As women's experience
is increasingly valued as a resource for developing knowledge, the resulting
values conflict with traditional views, and the new values will open avenues for
change.

SUMMARY OF EVOLVING DIRECTIONS IN NURSING THEORY

In the early 1950s, efforts to represent nursing theoretically produced broad
conceptualizations of nursing practice. These broad conceptual models or
frameworks (in our view, also theories) proliferated during the 1960s and
1970s and are growing and changing. These early theories represented an
ideal for nursing—the "oughts" of nursing. They suggested the nature of the
person, society and environment, and health; described the nurses' role and
the philosophic foundations of the profession; and challenged the reality of
nursing practice through their idealistic stance about nursing.

Although the broad conceptual models and frameworks were not typically developed using traditional scientific research processes, they did provide real direction for nursing by focusing on a general ideal of practice that
served as a guide for research and education. Table 3–6 presents a chrono-
logical list of nurse theorists who have produced broad conceptualizations of
nursing from the 1950s to the present. Many of the women who appear early
in the chronology continue to actively publish in the nursing literature. Some
of the nurse theorists listed later had a much earlier influence within nursing
by communicating their ideas in professional circles before they were published. The table also includes our view of the key emphasis of each theorist's
work. An interpretive summary of the writings of each theorist in the table can
be found in Appendix A.

Over time, the focus of these theories has changed significantly to parallel changes in society. Systems theory had widespread acceptance in the biologic and social sciences during the 1960s and its influence can be particularly

Table 3–6 Chronology of conceptual models in nursing (1952–1989)

Year of first major publication	Theorist	Key emphasis
1952	Hildegard E. Peplau	Interpersonal process is maturing force for personality.
1960	Faye G. Abedllah Irene L. Beland Almeda Martin Rugh V. Matheney	Patient's problems determine nursing care.
1961	Ida Jean Orlando	Interpersonal process alleviates distress.
1964	Ernestine Weidenbach	Helping process meets needs through art of individualizing care.
1966	Lydia E. Hall	Nursing care is person directed toward self-love.
1966	Joyce Travelbee	Meaning in illness determines how people respond.
1967	Myra E. Levine	Holism is maintained by conserving integrity.
1970	Martha E. Rogers	Person-environment are energy fields that evolve negentropically.
1971	Dorothea E. Orem	Self-care maintains wholeness.
1971	Imogene M. King	Transactions provide a frame of reference toward goal setting.
1974	Sr. Callista Roy	Stimuli disrupt an adaptive system.
1976	Josephine G. Paterson Loretta T. Zderad	Nursing is an existential experience of nurturing.
1978	Madeleine M. Leininger	Caring is universal and varies transculturally.
1979	Jean Watson	Caring is moral ideal: mind-body-soul engagement with another.
1979	Margaret A. Newman	Disease is a clue to preexisting life patterns.
1980	Dorothy E. Johnson	Subsystems exist in dynamic stability.
1981	Rosemarie Rizzo Parse	Indivisible beings and environment cocreate health.
1989	Patricia Benner and Judith Wrubel	Caring is central to the essence of nursing. It sets up what matters, enabling connection and concern. It creates possibility for mutual helpfulness.

noted in the work of Imogene King, Dorothy Johnson, and Sister Callista Roy. The theories of Martha Rogers, Rosemarie Parse, and Margaret Newman reflect theoretic perspectives in modern physics that move beyond earlier system concepts of equilibrium. Other theorists who continue to write also have changed their perspectives over time. These changes are often linked to changes in the social and political contexts within which nursing theories develop, and they reflect evolution of the theorist's ideas. Theorists whose perspective changes with successive publications include Sister Callista Roy, Jean Watson, and Madeleine Leininger.

These broad theories can be grouped according to some unique trait or feature. For example, Sisca-Riehl (1989) categorizes theories into developmental and interaction types, implying that these concepts are related to nursing. Common themes can also be seen in the influence of one theorist's ideas on others. Ernestine Weidenbach and Ida Jean Orlando both focus on the importance of meeting patient needs. Although from a different perspective, Leininger and Watson emphasize the concept of caring as a central focus for nursing. When theories are grouped, regardless of the category, central concepts or images for nursing are formed.

How theory is being defined and created in nursing is changing. With growing doctoral preparation, nurses are educated to conduct research and create theory, and the potential for creating theory based on and evolving from research increases.

Significant and valuable nursing theory at the midrange level is now being developed. Appendix B provides a summary of several examples of midrange theory and how they have been developed. Creating midrange theory relies on linking theory directly with research and with practice, or generating theory from practice-based research. In either approach, research, practice, and theory more readily interact to modify and shape all three dimensions. Whereas broad conceptual frameworks provide general ideals for practice, midrange theory can be used to more directly guide care.

Other major approaches to defining nursing have been developed and used but may not be identified as theory. Nursing diagnosis taxonomies are a prime example. The widespread recognition of nursing diagnoses represents the enactment of a theoretic position about nursing.

Theoretic activity is also increasing in relation to the ethical basis of nursing practice. Although early conceptual models and frameworks followed an empiric form of theory construction, they embodied normative goals that were grounded in an ethic of nursing. Within nursing, there is increasing recognition of the need to develop conceptualizations of ethics as ways of being rather than as sets of selectively applied rules and guidelines for practice.

CONCLUSION

In this chapter, we have presented an overview of the history from which theory in nursing evolves. The values and resources that influence theory development are rooted in history. The history of nursing determines the nature of nursing's knowledge and how knowledge in nursing develops. The history, values, and resources of nursing have been influenced by cultural and societal circumstances that closely parallel the status and role of women. As early theorists in nursing developed a sense of community and scholarship, they expressed differences and commonalities that have influenced more recent theoretic developments. A perspective of history and an understanding of values and resources affecting the development of theory make it possible to refine understandings of what theory is. In Chapter 4, we will examine various definitions of theory that have been published in nursing literature and develop a definition that is consistent with nursing's key concepts and patterns of knowing.

REFERENCES

Abdellah FG: The nature of nursing science, *Nurs Res* 18(5):390–93, 1969.

Abdellah FG et al: Patient-centered approaches to nursing, New York, 1960, The Macmillan Co.

Ashley JA: Hospitals, paternalism, and the role of the nurse, New York, 1976, Teacher's College Press.

Barnard KE and Neal MV: Maternal-child nursing research: review of the past and strategies for the future, *Nurs Res* 26(1):193–200, 1977.

Benner P: From novice to expert: excellence and power in clinical nursing practice, Menlo Park, 1984, Addison-Wesley.

Benner P: Quality of life: a phenomenological perspective on explanation, prediction, and understanding in nursing science, *Adv Nurs Sci* 8(1):1–14, 1985.

Benner P and Wrubel J: The primacy of caring, Menlo Park, 1989, Addision-Wesley.

Bramwell L: Use of life history in pattern identification and health promotion, *Adv Nurs Sci* 7(12):37–44, 1984.

Chinn PL and Wheeler CE: Feminism and nursing, *Nurs Outlook* 33(2):74–77, 1985.

Christy TE: Portrait of a leader, *Nurs Outlook* 6(6):72–75, 1969.

Dennis KE and Prescott PA: Florence Nightingale: yesterday, today, and tomorrow, *Adv Nurs Sci* 7(2):66–81, 1985.

Dickoff J and James P: A theory of theories: a position paper, *Nurs Res* 17(3):197–203, 1968.

Dickoff J and James P: Clarity to what end? *Nurs Res* 20(6):499–502, 1971.

Dickoff J, James P, and Wiedenbach E: Theory in a practice discipline. Part I:Practice-oriented theory, *Nurs Res* 17(5):415–35, 1968.

Donaldson SK and Crowley DM: The discipline of nursing, *Nurs Outlook* 26(2):113–20, 1978.

Ellis R: Commentary on "Toward a clearer understanding of the concept of nursing theory," *Nurs Res* 20(6):493–94, 1971.

Engel NS: On the vicissitudes of health appraisal, *Adv Nurs Sci* 7(1):12–23,1984.

Fawcett J: The relationship between theory and research: a double helix, *Adv Nurs Sci* 1(1):49–62, 1978.

Flaskerud JH and Halloran EJ: Areas of agreement in nursing theory development, *Adv Nurs Sci* 3(1):1–7, 1980.

Folta JR: Obfuscation or clarification: a reaction to Walker's concept of nursing theory, *Nurs Res* 20(6):496–99, 1971.

Francis G: Gesellshaft and the hospital: is total care a misnomer? *Adv Nurs Sci* 2(4):9–13, 1980.

Greenleaf NP: Sex-segregated occupations: relevance for nursing, *Adv Nurs Sci* 2(3):23–38, 1980.

Hall LE: A center for nursing, *Nurs Outlook* 11(11):805–6, 1963.

Hall LE: Nursing: what is it? *Can Nurse* 60(2):150–54, 1964.

Hall LE: Another view of nursing care and quality. In Straub KM and Parker KS, editors: Continuity in patient care: the role of nursing, Washington, DC, 1966, Catholic University Press, pp 47–60.

Hardy ME: Perspectives on nursing theory, *Adv Nurs Sci* 1(1):37–48, 1978.

Henderson V: The nature of nursing, *Am J Nurs* 64(8):62–68, 1964.

Henderson V: The nature of nursing, New York, 1966, The Macmillan Co.

Hughes L: The public image of the nurse, *Adv Nurs Sci* 2(3):55–72, 1980.

Jacobs, MK: Can nursing theory be tested? In Chinn PL, editor: Methodological issues in nursing, Rockville, 1986, Aspen Publications, Inc.

Johnson DE: The behavioral system model for nursing. In Riehl JP and Roy SR C, editors: Conceptual models for nursing practice, ed 2, New York, 1980, Appleton-Century-Crofts, pp 207–16.

Kalisch PA and Kalisch BJ: The advance of American nursing, Boston, 1978, Little, Brown, & Co.

Kelly LY: The nursing experience: Trends, challenges and transitions, ed 2, New York, 1992, The Macmillan Co.

King IM: Toward a theory for nursing: general concepts of human behavior, New York, 1971, John Wiley & Sons.

Kramer MK: Holistic nursing: implications for knowledge development and utilization. In Chaska NL: The nursing profession: turning points, St. Louis, 1990, Mosby-Year Book, Inc, pp 245–54.

Leininger MM: Doctoral programs for nurses: trends, questions, and projected plans, *Nurs Res* 25(3):201–10, 1976.

Leininger MM: Transcultural nursing: concepts theories and practices, New York, 1978, John Wiley & Sons.

Levine ME: The four conservation principles of nursing, *Nurs Forum* 6(1):93–98, 1967.

Lovell MC: The politics of medical deceptions: challenging the trajectory of history, *Adv Nurs Sci* 2:73–86, 1980.

Meleis AI: ReVisions in knowledge development: a passion for substance, *Scholarly Inquiry Nurs Pract* 1(1):5–19, 1987.

Melosh B: The physician's hand: work culture and conflict in American nursing, Philadelphia, 1982, Temple University Press.

Moccia, PA: A further investigation of "dialectical thinking as a means of understanding systems-in-development: relevance to Roger's principles," *Adv Nurs Sci* 7(4):33–38, 1985.

Moccia PA: A critique of compromise: beyond the methods debate, *Adv Nurs Sci* 10(4):1–9, 1988.

Newman MA: Theory development in nursing, Philadelphia, 1979, FA Davis Co.

Newman MA: Health as expanding consciousness, St. Louis, 1986, Mosby-Year Book, Inc.

Nightingale F: Notes on nursing: what it is and what it is not, New York, 1969, Dover Publications (unabridged republication of the first American Edition, as published in 1860 by D. Appleton and Co.).

Nightingale F: Cassandra, Old Westbury, NY, 1980, The Feminist Press (introduction by M. Stark and epilogue by C. MacDonald).

Orem DE: Nursing: concepts of practice, New York, 1971, McGraw-Hill Book Co, Inc.

Orlando IJ: The dynamic nurse-patient relationship: function, process, and principles, New York, 1961, GP Putnam's Sons (republished in 1990 by the National League for Nursing).

Parse RR: Man-living-health: a theory of nursing, New York, 1981, John Wiley & Sons.
Parse RR: Nursing science: major paradigms, theories and critiques, Philadelphia, 1987, WB Saunders.
Paterson JG and Zderad LT: Humanistic nursing, New York, 1976, John Wiley & Sons (republished in 1988 by National League for Nursing).
Peplau, HE: Interpersonal relations in nursing, New York, 1952, GP Putnam's Sons.
Reverby SM: Ordered to care: the dilemma of American nursing, 1850–1945, New York, 1987, Cambridge University Press.
Roberts S: Oppressed group behavior: implications for nursing, *Adv Nurs Sci* 5(4):21–30, 1983.
Rogers ME: An introduction to the theoretical basis of nursing, Philadelphia, 1970, FA Davis Co.
Roy, SR C: Introduction to nursing: an adaptation model, Englewood Cliffs, 1976, Prentice-Hall, Inc.
Sanger M: Margaret Sanger, an autobiography, New York, 1971, Dover Publications (originally published in 1938 by WW Norton).
Silverstein NG: Lillian Wald at Henry Street, 1893–1895, *Adv Nurs Sci* 7(2):1–12, 1985.
Sisca-Riehl JP, editor: Conceptual models for nursing practice, ed 3, New York, 1989, Appleton-Lange.
Smith JA: The idea of health: implications for the nursing professional, New York, 1983, Teachers College Press.
Stevens PE: A critical social reconceptualization of environment in nursing: implications for methodology, *Adv Nurs Sci* 11(4):56–68, 1989.
Tooley SA: The life of Florence Nightingale, New York, 1905, The Macmillan Co.
Travelbee J: Interpersonal aspects of nursing, Philadelphia, 1966, FA Davis Co.
Travelbee J: Interpersonal aspects of nursing, ed 2, Philadelphia, 1971, FA Davis Co.
Wald LD: The house of Henry Street, New York, 1971, Dover Publications, (originally published in 1915 by Holt, Rinehart, and Winston, Inc).
Walker, LO: Toward a clearer understanding of the concept of nursing theory, *Nurs Res* 20(5):428–35, 1971.
Walker LO: Rejoinder to commentary: toward a clearer understanding of the concept of nursing theory, *Nurs Res* 21(1):59–62, 1972.
Watson J: Nursing: the philosophy and science of caring, Boston, 1979, Little, Brown, & Co (republished in 1988 by the National League for Nursing).
Watson J: Nursing: human science and human care, Norwalk, CT 1985, Appleton-Century-Crofts.
Whall AL: Congruence between existing theories of family functioning and nursing theories, *Adv Nurs Sci* 3(1):59–67, 1980.
Wheeler CE: The American Journal of Nursing and the socialization of a profession, 1900–1920, *Adv Nurs Sci* 7(2):20–34, 1985.
Wiedenbach E: Clinical nursing: a helping art, New York, 1964, Springer Publishing Co, Inc.
Winstead-Fry P: The scientific method and its impact on holistic health, *Adv Nurs Sci* 2(4):1–7, 1980.
Woodham-Smith C: Florence Nightingale: 1820–1910, New York, 1983, Atheneum.
Wooldridge PJ: Meta-theories of nursing: a commentary on Dr. Walker's article, *Nurs Res* 20(6):494–95, 1971.
Yura H and Torres G: Today's conceptual frameworks within baccalaureate nursing programs, Faculty Curriculum Development, Part III, New York, 1975, National League for Nursing.

4

Nursing theory: an examination of the concept

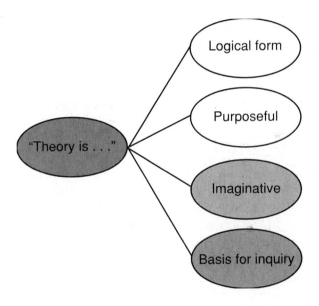

The word *theory* has many meanings. From our perspective, nursing theory need not focus on any one purpose or trait of theory. A definition that is useful for characterizing nursing theory is broad enough to incorporate and encourage diverse types of theory.

What exactly is nursing theory? There are several ways to answer this seemingly simple question. In Chapters 1 and 2, we reviewed the dimensions and forms of empirically patterned knowledge and discussed a broad definition of theory, which provided a general understanding of the nature of theory and its contribution to the whole of knowing. In this chapter, we examine four distinct definitions of theory and a range of traits that characterize theory. From this, we propose a definition of theory that is sufficiently broad to include many types of theory yet sufficiently specific to differentiate empiric theory from other forms of scholarly discourse. Our definition reflects the range of theory development processes and outcomes that we believe are necessary for the growth of nursing knowledge.

COMPLEXITY OF ABSTRACT CONCEPTS

The word *theory* has multiple meanings because it represents a very abstract concept. Since theory is also built from concepts, we begin this discussion of what theory is by considering the nature of concepts.

We define a concept as a complex mental formulation of experience. All concepts can be located on a continuum from the empiric (more directly experienced) to the abstract (more mentally constructed) (Jacox, 1974; Kaplan, 1964). In one sense, all concepts are both empiric and abstract. They are empiric because they are formed from encounters with perceptible reality. They are abstract because they are cognitive representations of what is perceptually experienced. Concepts differ in the ways in which they directly relate to perceptible reality. Some concepts are formed from very direct experiences with reality, whereas others are formed from indirect experiences. Figure 4–1 illustrates this continuum. Relatively empiric concepts are ideas that are formed from direct observations of objects, properties, or events. As concepts become more abstract, they can only be experienced indirectly. The most abstract concepts encompass a complex network of subconcepts that can only be inferred. Concepts formed about objects such as a cup or properties such as hot are examples of highly empiric concepts because the object or property that represents the idea (empiric indicator) can be directly experienced through the senses. A relatively empiric property such as biological sex can also be observed directly by noting the primary and secondary sexual characteristics that identify a person as male or female. Properties such as height and weight can be measured using standardized instruments. Since the measurement is relatively direct, height and weight are empiric concepts.

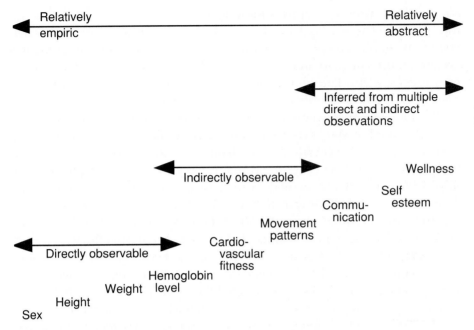

FIGURE 4–1   Example of empiric-abstract continuum.

As concepts become more abstract, their reality basis and their empiric indicators become less concrete and less directly measurable. Assessment of an abstract concept depends increasingly on indirect means. Although an indirect assessment or observation is different from direct measurement, it is considered to be a reasonable indicator of the concept. Hemoglobin level is representative of a concept that cannot be directly observed but can be indirectly seen with the aid of laboratory instruments. This type of measurement depends on more complex and less direct forms of instrumentation.

Cardiovascular fitness is an example of a concept that is midrange on the empiric-abstract continuum. Concepts increase in complexity in this range, and several empiric indicators must be assessed. Because no object such as cardiovascular fitness exists, a definition is required if we are to know what it is. Even though definitions for less empirically based concepts are thoughtfully formulated, they are arbitrary, because many different definitions could be chosen. As concepts become increasingly abstract, definitions become more dependent on the theoretic meaning of the concept and the purpose for defining it.

Self-esteem is an example of a highly abstract concept for which there are no direct measures. The instruments or tools that are developed to assess self-esteem depend on theoretic definitions serving a specific purpose and are built on multiple behavioral responses that experts agree are associated with that concept. Ideas about these responses may be derived from a theory or may generate from concept clarification (see Chapter 5). Each behavioral trait contained in the tool can be considered as partial indicators of self-esteem. When the composite behaviors are built into an assessment tool, it is usually a more adequate indicator for the abstract concept than any one behavior taken alone. The composite score obtained from the tool is then considered to be a measurement constructed as an empiric indicator.

Highly abstract concepts are sometimes called constructs. Constructs are the most complex type of concept on the empiric-abstract continuum. These concepts include ideas with a reality base so abstract that it is constructed from multiple sources of direct and indirect evidence. An example of a construct is wellness. While the idea of wellness exists, it cannot be directly observed. Figure 4–1 illustrates the idea that highly abstract concepts are constructed from other concepts. All of the concepts shown on the continuum (as well as others) can be included in the concept of wellness.

Some abstract concepts have little meaning outside the context of a theory. For example, Levine (1967) coined the word *trophicogenic* to mean "nurse-induced illness." Rogers (1970) discussed three "principles of homeodynamics." Rogers' term *homeodynamics* is a combination of the Latin root word *homeo* meaning "similar to" or "like" and the common English term *dynamics*, meaning "pattern of change or growth." The reader can infer the meaning "change processes" for the term *homeodynamics*, which is consistent with Rogers' intent.

Abstract concepts may also acquire additional meaning through gradual transfer into common language usage. Freud's concept of *ego* is an example. Once the word *ego* had no common meaning outside of Freud's theory, but today, with gradual changes in its meaning and broad usage outside the theory, everyone knows the meaning of "a big ego."

Although it is usually not necessary or possible to identify precisely where concepts fit on an empiric-abstract continuum, it is important to understand that concepts vary in the degree to which they are connected to empiric reality and the extent to which their meaning is mentally constructed.

Defining and understanding concepts

When you begin to study an abstract concept like theory, it is natural to wonder why it is difficult to grasp the meaning of the term and understand the concept. It is helpful to recognize that even highly empiric concepts like cup are not easily understood and defined. To illustrate, conjure an image of a cup. What you have done is create an image of the object in your mind—you have brought into awareness a concept. Now describe the image you have in your mind's eye. Your definition might be something like this:

> **cup**   A hard-surfaced, hollow cylinder, closed on one end, with a small handle attached to the cylindric surface, that is often used for drinking.

Note that the cup defined above is for drinking, but other cup images are possible, as illustrated in the phrases "to cup my hand," "to offer a cup of cheer," and "the golf ball dropped into the cup." When these different meanings for cup are suggested, where you would place the concept on the empiric-abstract continuum changes. Placing a concept on the continuum requires that you know its definition or how it is being used. A "cup of cheer," unlike the drinking cup, cannot be directly experienced but can be inferred from behaviors that differ across cultural contexts. The use of the word *cup* as in "a cup of cheer" represents a more abstract concept than use of the word in reference to an ordinary drinking cup.

In the development of language, once a word representing an object has been established, the object may change, and ambiguity develops about the use of the term. For example, the term *cup* can be used to refer to a stoneware mug or a china teacup. Each object is quite different, and they are found in different social contexts, but the definition given above for each is adequate. To differentiate two types of cups, the definition would need to include additional features of the cup that are appropriate to the context in which it is used, material that the cup is made of, or other objects that accompany the use of the cup.

To further illustrate the difficulty of defining even concrete concepts, omit the handle from the original definition of cup. The definition now reads:

cup A hard-surfaced, hollow cylinder closed on one end, often used for drinking.

You can now appreciate the significance of the handle for distinguishing this object from a drinking glass. When this portion of the definition is omitted, the dimensions and composition of the object, as well as the context of usage, become important for determining whether the object is a cup or a glass. A cup may be defined as being shorter and wider than a glass, and differentiation between them would rely on their physical dimensions.

Sometimes distinctions between objects are not important, and a definition that includes a wide range of meaning is adequate. Now imagine an opaque, styrofoam drinking vessel that holds about 8 ounces, has no handle, is shaped like a section of a cone, and is closed on the narrow end. Is this object a cup or a glass? For some people, it is a cup, for others a glass, and for still others it is both! Without detailed definitions for both the concepts of cup and glass, there is no basis for distinguishing between the two, and, even with definitions, the decision about which label to use is arbitrary and depends on the purpose.

Ambiguities in definitions

Ambiguities exist in all definitions, even for those of very concrete realities. It is difficult, if not impossible, to construct a precise definition. For example, our definition of the word *cup* does not specify how or where the handle is placed on the cylindric surface. These ambiguities are greatly magnified when defining highly abstract concepts. Defining abstract realities requires a tolerance of ambiguity. Rather than try to fix ambiguities, choices are made about which empiric reality is represented in an abstract concept and which is not.

Because of its highly abstract nature, the word *theory* is defined in many different ways. The question, Is this a theory or a conceptual framework? often arises. This question is reasonable, for one nurse's theory may be another's conceptual framework. Reasonable definitions are neither right nor wrong, and it may be difficult to decide about the best definition for a given purpose. Authors use these words differently; most authors provide the reader either explicit definitions or explanations on which their usage is based. Generally, conceptual frameworks refer to a logical grouping of related theories. Models are generally fairly concrete representations of relationships and are often used within theories to illustrate relationships and structures within theories. Models may also be used as heuristic devices used to guide theory testing, so any one theory could be modeled differently for different purposes. Our aim is to present various definitions of the highly abstract concept of theory, examine them for commonalties and differences, and present a definition for the term *theory* that is suited to our ideas about how theory develops in nursing.

COMPARATIVE ANALYSIS OF DEFINITIONS OF THEORY

In Chapter 2, we defined theory broadly as a "systematic abstraction of reality that serves some purpose." Theoretic purposes included the description, explanation, and prediction of empiric reality. Although this definition is not incorrect, it is very broad and therefore not always helpful in understanding what theory is and how it is created. The phrase "systematic abstraction" suggests a product or outcome, as well as a series of thoughts, actions, or processes by which the outcomes are created. The definitions we examine here suggest the specific processes that are used to create the systematic abstraction that is theory. The definitions also suggest different possible outcomes when theory development processes are carried out.

Rose McKay: The form of theory development

Theory has been defined by McKay as a "logically interconnected set of confirmed hypotheses" (McKay, 1969, p. 394). This definition implies that reasoned thought, armchair style, that does not use confirmed hypotheses as raw material will not produce theory. The definition also implies that research processes are integral to the building of theory because confirmed hypotheses do not arise otherwise. Using McKay's definition, a conceptual framework or model would refer to writings that reflect conceptual relationships that are not yet confirmed or tested, reserving the term *theory* only for interconnected relationships that have been tested.

A hypothesis is a type of propositional statement. It is a single statement of a proposed relationship between two or more variables. Hypotheses can take several forms and still provide a basis for developing theory. A neutral hypothesis asserts that one variable (X) is related to a second variable (Y) or that one variable (X) changes in relation to another (Y) without indicating the direction of change. A directional hypothesis indicates the direction of association between variables where, as one variable (X) increases or decreases, a second (Y) also increases or decreases.

A confirmed hypothesis is a relationship statement for which there is research support. It can be either directional or neutral. Hypothesis testing requires that certain controls and procedures be adhered to and that statistical models be applied in the confirmation process. Thus, a specific type of research is basic to the development of theory according to this definition of theory.

Most theory in nursing does not meet the requirements of the McKay definition, yet the definition is not wrong. In fact, it reflects a traditional notion of what theory is, particularly within the natural sciences (physics, chemistry, biology). In sciences in which phenomena obey natural laws or can be isolated from their context and controlled, it is possible to confirm hypotheses and logically interconnect them to create theory. In such sciences, the range of variables is often narrow, and experimental research approaches are used so variables can be singularly added in a controlled environment and their effects on outcomes can be monitored. Control over the environment and the variables under study helps ensure that a hypothesis will be reliably confirmed or rejected.

In addition to requiring confirmed hypotheses for theory construction, the McKay definition implies that the hypotheses are connected using rules of logic. The logic may be either deductive or inductive. The following sections provide an overview of each of these forms of logic.

Deductive forms of logic. Deductive logic is a system of reasoning in which propositions—assertions of relationship—are interrelated in a consistent way. In deductive logic, the logician begins with two premises as propositions (sometimes called axioms) and draws a conclusion, or a proposition, that is directly dependent on the premises. In logic, the format used is fixed. Format refers to the structure of interrelationships among the premises and the conclusion without regard to the meaningfulness of the premises. It is possible to have a valid, or formally correct, logical argument that is not meaningful when compared with empiric experience.

Theory developed from application of deductive systems of logic is only as sound as the premises on which the argument is based. One form of deductive logic is

(premise) A is B.
(premise) C is A.
(conclusion) C is B.

The problem of reaching a sound conclusion occurs when concepts, representing human characteristics, are substituted for the letters. The problem of soundness of deductive logic can be illustrated with the following:

(premise) Humans (A) use cups with handles (B).
(premise) Infants (C) are humans (A).
(conclusion) Infants (C) use cups with handles (B).

With substitutions of words representing selected concepts, the soundness of the conclusion is questionable, even though the form is valid. In this example, the conclusion that infants use cups with handles cannot be justified as being consistent with empiric experience.

Confirmed hypotheses as premises are grounded in empiric reality. Because they are tested by research standards with imposed limitations, they can be considered valid. Confirmed hypotheses hold more potential for sound conclusions than unconfirmed hypotheses or suppositions. An example of a deductive argument in valid form and with reasonable premises (though unconfirmed) follows:

(premise) Pregnant mammals retain fluid.
(premise) Pregnant women are pregnant mammals.
(conclusion) Pregnant women retain fluid.

The form of the argument is valid, and the first premise could be confirmed by research. Assuming confirmation of the first premise and the valid analytic (true by definition) nature of the second, the conclusion is likely to be more sound than one generated from untested premises.

Deductive logic is a way of reasoning. Its rules require a valid form of interrelationships between statements. Two or more relational statements are used to draw a concluding relational statement or proposition. A proposition, meaning an assertion of relationship between variables, can also be called a theorem. Premises, the statements on which the conclusion is based, may also be called hypotheses, suppositions, axioms, or simply propositions.

Laws may also arise from the application of deductive logic, especially in mathematics. A law represents a highly generalizable assertion of relationship between variables. Laws can also be derived using inductive forms of logical thought.

Terms other than *axiom* and *theorem* for *premises* and *conclusions* in the empiric sciences (sciences other than logic and mathematics) reflect the tentative nature of propositions. In the empiric sciences, premises and conclusions may be called hypotheses or suppositions, implying that they are still open to challenge.

Deductive conclusions can be used as premises in progressive logical arguments. This process links one logical idea to another, forming a type of theory. McKay's definition of theory limits theory to relationships that are confirmed research hypotheses. Some theory, however, develops by linking logical statements, which is known as deducing hypotheses, implying that the theoretic relationships have not necessarily been confirmed empirically.

Although deductive systems of logic are valuable, there are certain hazards. *limits* Deduction based on suppositions or unconfirmed hypotheses may result in an unsound argument that seems reasonable at face value. When the soundness of a conclusion is unknown, it may be erroneously assumed to be sound without serious challenge, especially if it seems reasonable. Deductive arguments based on confirmed hypotheses have a greater likelihood of achieving soundness, at least within the limits of their research testing. Although the empiric soundness of any conclusion may never be finally known, the utility of logical deductive conclusions for nursing increases if the premises have a degree of confirmation.

Inductive forms of logic.   In the traditional view of science, deductive logic is the predominant form used in producing theory. However, the logical interconnections could also arise from the application of a second common system of logic: the inductive mode. This approach to theory development is being used in nursing in such approaches as grounded theory (Glaser and Strauss, 1967). In inductive logic, the reasoning method relies on observing multiple particular instances and then combining those particulars into a larger whole. This can occur when the particular instances observed share common features and are part of a larger set of phenomena. The following example illustrates this approach: Assume that X1, X2, ... X5 are unique instances of a larger set Y and that Y is associated with an effect or characteristic Z. The reasoning used is

> X1 is a member of set Y and is associated with Z.
> X2 is a member of set Y and is associated with Z.
> X3 is a member of set Y and is associated with Z.
> X4 is a member of set Y and is associated with Z.
> X5 is a member of set Y and is associated with Z.

Therefore X6, X7, . . . Xn, or all X's, are members of set Y, and are associated with Z.

To substitute an empiric experience for the letter symbols in this illustration, let X be specific surgical techniques, let Y be surgical intervention, and let Z be postoperative pain. With these substitutions, the argument would proceed in the following manner:

> A dilatation and curettage is a surgical intervention associated with postoperative pain.
> A laparotomy is a surgical intervention associated with postoperative pain.
> A laser ablation is a surgical intervention associated with postoperative pain.
> A burr hole is a surgical intervention associated with postoperative pain.
> A closed reduction is a surgical intervention associated with postoperative pain.
> Therefore, all surgical interventions are associated with postoperative pain.

In this example, the reasoning is that many specific instances of surgical techniques as surgical interventions are associated with the concept of postoperative pain. These surgical techniques share the empiric feature of being surgical interventions, which in turn are associated with postoperative pain.

Inductive reasoning would be considered sound when all specific instances of surgical techniques as surgical intervention (in our example, X's) were observed to be associated with postoperative pain. A conclusion is drawn from the observation of specific instances of X's as subsets of surgical intervention associated with pain, and, when observations have been exhausted, the sets X and Y merge, and the argument is sound.

A second example illustrates some pitfalls of inductive reasoning. In this example, birds such as crows and ravens (X's) are specific instances of a larger set black birds (Y), and Z is having the ability to fly. The example is

> A crow is a black bird that can fly.
> A raven is a black bird that can fly.
> A starling is a black bird that can fly.
> A grackle is a black bird that can fly.
> A vulture is a black bird that can fly.
> Therefore, all black birds can fly.

Since it is not possible to observe all instances of black birds that can fly, there is the possibility that the instance of a black bird that cannot fly will be missed. For example, if you chance to observe a black ostrich, your conclusion must be revised to accommodate the instance of a black bird that cannot fly.

Inductive logic is limited because it is not possible to observe all instances of a specific event. This limitation must be considered when using inductive logic to generate theory.

In the example of surgical techniques as surgical interventions associated with pain, assume that the five instances cited were confirmed to be associated with postoperative pain. In inductive logic, useful theory can be developed from observing and confirming that additional specific instances of surgical intervention were also associated with pain and concluding that all surgical interventions result in postoperative pain. It is not practical to show that all instances of surgical techniques as surgical intervention are associated with pain. The association can be shown to a degree of probability sufficient to develop useful theory, particularly when the context is limited.

Comparison of induction and deduction.   Deductive logic is reasoning from the general to the particular. Inductive logic is reasoning from the particular to the general. In inductive logic, particular instances are observed to be consistently part of a larger whole or set, and the set of particular instances is merged with that larger whole. This larger set can then be considered in relation to still another set of events or phenomena in another logical system.

In deductive logic, the premises as starting points embody two variables that can be categorized in relation to each other as broad or specific. In the one example, pregnant mammals (a broad concept) were said to retain fluid (a specific concept). In the other premise, pregnant women were said to be pregnant mammals; that is, pregnant women were specifically members of a broader class (pregnant mammals). The conclusion contains both of the specific variables: pregnant women retain fluid. In deductive logic, the movement is from premises embodying broad and specific variables to a conclusion in which the variables are more specific.

Like most other words, deduction and induction have common meanings related to, but different from, their meaning within systems of logic. People often state that they deduce hypotheses from theory or deductively develop theory. These deductions are not the result of applying rules of logic but arise out of careful thought without specifically using a system of logic. Used like this, deduction implies that a more general theory was a source of specific hypotheses or relational statements.

With induction, people induce hypotheses and relationships by observing or experiencing an empiric reality and reaching some conclusion. These related meanings of induction and deduction should be noted because sometimes the terms refer to systems of logic and to rules and conventions for the ordering of reasoning. At other times, the terms refer to a general approach to thinking, short of logical rules but similar in form.

McKay's definition of theory is useful because it focuses on the significance of logical thought and empiric confirmation in developing some forms of theory. However, as McKay notes, other definitions of theory that require less stringency in their approach are needed in nursing. Flexible approaches to theory development are valuable because nursing empirics must be consistent with the assumptions of human science. Nursing deals with a wide range of events that are complex and interconnected with countless other events. A strict and singular use of rules of logic and traditional scientific empiric confirmation is not consistent with nursing's concern with holistic beings whose actions are not totally governed by natural laws.

James Dickoff and Patricia James: The outcome of theory

Dickoff and James (1968, p. 198) propose a definition of theory quite different from that of McKay. They define theory as "a conceptual system or framework invented to some purpose." Using their broad definition, you could include conceptual framework or model as a theory. Nursing is a service profession that has the promotion of health as one of its goals. Dickoff and James state that nursing must generate theory that will achieve its goals or purposes. In this definition, *purpose* is a key word, since theory is purpose-oriented. In McKay's definition, even though clinical purpose is not explicitly addressed, some purpose—for example, explanation or prediction—would be identifiable for theory that is derived from research-tested hypotheses. Dickoff and James' definition, requires the explicit articulation of a clear purpose or goal that directs the entire theory building effort (Dickoff and James, 1968; Dickoff, James, and Wiedenbach, 1968).

Invention is a second key idea within the Dickoff and James definition of theory. Invention implies that nursing creates the abstraction of reality that will achieve its purpose. The abstraction that is theory must be fashioned or made to happen, and its creation cannot occur apart from purpose. An analogy of a motor trip from the West Coast to the eastern seaboard will illustrate this point. If you are in California and only know you want to move by car, you can get into the car and drive, and you will go somewhere. When you do this—get into a car and drive—you are only able to retrospectively describe a route taken. If you decide on a destination before beginning, you can invent and create the route as you proceed. One choice would be to take more time and wander around on the side roads and gather a lot of detailed experiences. Another choice would be to travel quickly on the interstate highway, gathering only those experiences that can be gleaned from the narrow vista. Your choice would be influenced by the amount of time and resources you have, the amount of detail you want or need, and your personal preference. According to Dickoff and James, theory building is a process of creating and inventing the pathway from among alternate choices; your choice is guided by your destination and the context in which you are making the choice. If there is no destination, it is only possible to give a retrospective account of features of the route. The Dickoff and James definition requires that a goal be stated and the way toward it created. Theory is deliberately created to achieve a purpose, and that purpose is value-laden.

When theory is invented with some purpose in mind, theory development will occur in a way that is related to that purpose. Using this definition, the general form taken is a conceptual framework, and the processes of abstraction are varied. *Conceptual* means "of or pertaining to concepts," whereas *framework* implies features of a structure or network. A conceptual framework is a network or structure of empirically based abstractions (concepts) that are represented by word symbols.

For Dickoff and James, theory exists on four levels: factor-isolating, factor-relating (also called situation-depicting), situation-relating, and situation-producing (Dickoff and James, 1968; Dickoff, James, and Wiedenbach, 1968). Level 1, factor-isolating, involves the naming or classification of phenomena. Level 2, factor-relating, implies correlating or associating factors in such a way that they become part of larger units that meaningfully depict a situation. Level 3, situation- relating, explains and predicts how situations are related. Level 4, situation-producing, requires sufficient knowledge about how and why situations are related so that, using theory as a guide, differing but valued situations can be produced (Dickoff and James, 1968, p. 200). Writings that can be categorized at each of the four levels are considered theory.

For Dickoff, James, and Wiedenbach (1968), the three ingredients of situation-producing theory (level 4) are (1) goal content, (2) prescriptions, and (3) survey list. The goal content conveys the purpose, whereas prescriptions and survey list compose the major part of the conceptual framework. Prescriptions are specific directives for care that can be demonstrated to be effective in achieving the desired outcomes. The invention involves devising and interrelating the conceptual framework components of prescriptions and survey list to achieve the purpose.

McKay's definition also implies the notion of level change as theory builds. If induction is the logical process used to build theory, theoretic levels change as concepts merge and become more inclusive. Deduction processes affect the level of theory by generating more particular knowledge as the logic proceeds. In contrast, for Dickoff and James the level of development does not necessarily relate to breadth of concepts, but classification of the level occurs according to how theoretic content builds to achieve the stated goal. According to Dickoff and James, research can be included in the theory development process. Although Dickoff and James imply that theory development progresses through four levels, all nursing efforts need not start at level 1. Whether implicit or explicit, theory at the situation-producing level builds on theory developed at lower levels.

In their definition, Dickoff and James use the phrase "conceptual framework." This includes as theory a wide variety of systematic abstractions developed by a variety of means and with varying precision. The survey list is an organized, empirically grounded guide to achieving a purpose. It assumes that prescriptions can never be complete. Survey lists embellish the prescriptions and aid goal achievement. The survey list is developed systematically using methods that are different from confirming hypotheses. Dickoff and James' requirement that an explicit clinical purpose be achieved differs from other definitions of theory. To Dickoff and James, situation-producing theory is essential in nursing; a clinical purpose must be clearly stated. Once the goal is determined and communicated, nurses then invent or create the path to the goal. Specific goal content increases the likelihood that descriptions, explanations, and predictions will be useful in nursing practice. Naming the goal content promotes theory development, which is clearly within nursing's area of concern and demystifies the theory development enterprise.

Jean Watson: The tentative nature of theory

Watson (1985, p. 1) defines theory as "An imaginative grouping of knowledge, ideas, and experience that are represented symbolically and seek to illuminate a given phenomena." Watson's purpose for theory—"seek[ing] to illuminate a given phenomena"—implies a broad set of purposes for theory that could include understanding, describing, explaining, and predicting nursing phenomena. This implies that the nurse can use theory to project and work toward goals. Using Watson's definition, some scholarly writings would be excluded as theory if they lack the creative or imaginative element; these writings might be more appropriately called conceptual frameworks or models because they pictorially or linguistically arise from images of "what is." Theory, using Watson's definition, arises from the imagination and creativity of the theorist, implying that the theory challenges existing assumptions about "what is" and links or blends knowledge, ideas, and experience in a creative way.

Dickoff and James, by contrast, emphasize a specific practice goal as central to theory, with the concepts of the theory organized in such a way that goal achievement is explained. McKay's definition implies a general theoretic purpose.

Because theory illuminates a given phenomena, Watson suggests that theory is bounded and limited. The phrases "seek to illuminate" and "imaginative grouping" are important in this definition because they make explicit the nature of theory as a tentative creation. The fact that theory is tentative is often implied in major writings on the subject but is seldom directly acknowledged. The tentativeness of theory may not be obvious, because myths about theory perpetuate the notion that theory is somewhat final; since theory represents empiric reality, it is assumed to be reality. Science is grounded in a traditional view that truths exist independently from their discoverers. Discovered truths are assumed to proceed toward some ultimate and unchanging final truth. Consistent with emerging views, theory, research, and traditional science are no longer thought to hold claim on eternal truths. Although theory may be a valuable representation of empiric experience, it is not final; it is tentative.

In Watson's definition, the phrase "represented symbolically" is important because theory is a mediated (representational) form of knowledge. Mediated knowledge is conveyed through the use of symbols or words. For Watson, "knowledge, ideas, and experience" are represented symbolically as theory, integrating personal values, perspective, and biases of the theorist. Watson's definition of theory gives credence to personal ideas and experiences of nurses as valuable sources of knowledge.

Rosemary Ellis: Theory as a guide for inquiry

Ellis' (1968, p. 217) definition of theory is "conceptual and pragmatic principles forming a general frame of reference for a field of inquiry." This definition of theory provides a reference point for guiding research, inquiry, and practice with assumed links between the two. Although not explicit in the definition, for Ellis a purpose of theory could be to achieve clinical goals, since theory provides a reference point for guiding a field of inquiry. According to Ellis, if nursing practice provides the focus of inquiry, theory could help achieve a clinical purpose in the manner proposed by Dickoff and James. The wording of Ellis' definition suggests that research and theory are closely interrelated.

According to this definition, principles composing theory form a conceptual framework that may or may not have strict logical interconnections. Theory as a means to guide inquiry implies that concepts are defined or used with a particular meaning, that certain assumptions are articulated, and that goals exist. This definition complements the other definitions with the idea that theory can function to deliberately guide research and inquiry. Using this definition, what might be called a conceptual framework or model by some could be called theory, as long as the ideas are useful to guide inquiry.

A COMPREHENSIVE DEFINITION OF THEORY FOR NURSING

Although the preceding definitions are different, they share common features. Collectively, they define a wide range of functions for theory. All are legitimate and accepted; each one focuses on a possible dimension of meaning. The four definitions are

1. A logically interconnected set of confirmed hypotheses (McKay, 1969)
2. A conceptual system or framework invented to some purpose (Dickoff and James, 1968)

3. An imaginative grouping of knowledge, ideas, and experience that are represented symbolically and seek to illuminate a given phenomenon (Watson, 1985)
4. Conceptual and pragmatic principles forming a general frame of reference for a field of inquiry (Ellis, 1968)

Beliefs about the nature of theory arise in part from the various fields of inquiry from which nursing knowledge is developed. Some nursing theorists come from educational traditions in which the ideal of theory is logically linked sets of confirmed hypotheses. Others were educated in disciplines in which theory is viewed as loosely connected hypothetic conjectures. In other disciplines, theory is viewed as philosophically based sets of beliefs and values about human nature and action. In some of the disciplines, little viable theory exists. As a result, the nursing literature contains varying definitions for theory, but this diversity only serves to stimulate further understanding and development of theory.

From our perspective, nursing theory need not be limited to any one theoretic form. A definition that is useful for characterizing nursing theory must be broad enough to include diverse theory types. Our definition of theory is

theory   A creative and rigorous structuring of ideas that project a tentative, purposeful, and systematic view of phenomena.

Using our definition, all theory comprises a creative and rigorous structuring of ideas. The ideas are structured as concepts and represented by word symbols. In order for theory to project a systematic view of phenomena, the concepts contained within the theory must be conveyed within relationship statements and defined within the context of the theory. In theorizing, the theorist creates a language and structure that imparts to theory its systematic nature. Theory is purposive; theorists create theory for some reason. The purpose may take many forms. Theory is tentative and thus is grounded in assumptions, value choices, and the creative and imaginative judgment of the theorist.

Using our definition, differentiating theory as a form that is distinct from conceptual framework or model is similar to the differentiation that comes from Watson's definition. Our definition requires mental creativity reflected in the structure that moves beyond simply depicting "what is."

Figure 4–2 summarizes key phrases from the four definitions we have examined and shows how these phrases relate to the definition we have synthesized. We show the major characteristics and structural traits of theory that are suggested by our definition of theory. The four definitions we examined were selected to focus on certain characteristics of theory that are consistent with the concept of theory, but none of the previous definitions address all of those characteristics. The definition we have synthesized incorporates a wide range of methods or forms for the development of theory and represents theory as both

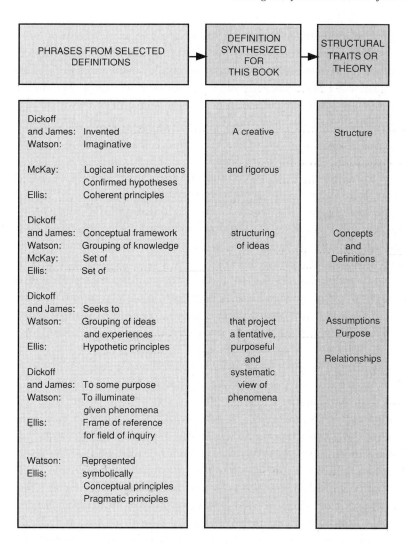

PHRASES FROM SELECTED DEFINITIONS		DEFINITION SYNTHESIZED FOR THIS BOOK	STRUCTURAL TRAITS OR THEORY
Dickoff and James:	Invented	A creative	Structure
Watson:	Imaginative		
McKay:	Logical interconnections Confirmed hypotheses	and rigorous	
Ellis:	Coherent principles		
Dickoff and James:	Conceptual framework	structuring of ideas	Concepts and Definitions
Watson:	Grouping of knowledge		
McKay:	Set of		
Ellis:	Set of		
Dickoff and James:	Seeks to		Assumptions Purpose
Watson:	Grouping of ideas and experiences	that project a tentative, purposeful and	
Ellis:	Hypothetic principles		Relationships
Dickoff and James:	To some purpose	systematic view of phenomena	
Watson:	To illuminate given phenomena		
Ellis:	Frame of reference for field of inquiry		
Watson:	Represented		
Ellis:	symbolically Conceptual principles Pragmatic principles		

FIGURE 4–2   Interrelationships between definitions and features of theory.

process and product. These characteristics of theory provide the basis for determining components used to describe theory that are presented in Chapter 6.

DEFINITIONS OF TERMS RELATED TO THEORY

Once a definition of theory is created, it is possible to analyze how theory differs from related terms such as *science, philosophy, paradigm,* and *model.* Like the word *theory,* these terms are highly abstract and have multiple meanings. In order to resolve differences between similar, yet different terms such as *conceptual frame-work* and *theory*, definitions of both can be created. It is possible to arrive at defi-nitions for different terms that are alike, and it is equally possible that definitions for the same term will reflect fundamental differences in meaning. The defini-tions of related terms—like our definition of theory—may not be universally ac-cepted, but we believe that they are reasonable and reflect common meanings.

Science

Science is both an approach to the generation of knowledge and the results of using that approach. Science—the process—uses methods that are valid and re-liable within a defined area of concern. These methods include different ap-proaches to research, as well as critical and logical thought. Science is also a body of knowledge; that is, it is the facts, theories, and descriptions generated when using empiric processes of science. The processes of science create systematic representations of reality that are accessible to the human senses and are there-fore called empiric. When we use the term *empirics* as a pattern of knowing, we imply that the pattern depends on accessible sensory experience to create knowl-edge and form understanding. From this perspective, empirics can include but does not require strict adherence to the tenets of traditional science.

Traditional natural science structures empiric knowledge without con-cern for the intentions of the person or the meaning of behavior. Natural sci-ence assumes that the scientist and the object of study are separate and that what is being studied is governed by laws and rules that do not vary. Discovering these laws and rules makes it possible to predict and subsequently control. In this view, the proper procedures of science assume that the scien-tist's behavior and values do not influence the discovery of knowledge.

Human science approaches draw on the traditions of natural science. These sciences differ in that empiric knowledge development must account for the thinking, feeling, and intentional characteristics of human nature. Because of this, scholars working in the human sciences have begun to develop methods that acknowledge the intimate connection between the scientist and what is stud-ied. The shifts in the assumptions, processes, and outcomes for traditional sci-ence that have emerged from the human science perspective are reflected in our approach to theory and knowledge development in nursing. This includes a shift toward understanding rather than prediction, as well as a rejection of the tradi-tional view of control as being neither desirable or possible.

Philosophy

Philosophy is a form of disciplined inquiry that discerns general traits of real-ity and sets forth rationale on which value principles rest, including principles of goodness, justness, duty, and fairness. Philosophy deals with many phenomena that are not suitable for empiric study and contains many branches of thought, each with its own theories. Competing explanations about the nature of reality can exist within the discipline of philosophy. Knowledge development in nursing rests on basic philosophic tenets and assumptions that are derived from selected schools of philosophic thought, including theories about the nature of reality, the nature of knowledge and knowing, ways of discerning reality, and principles of value.

Research

Research is application of formalized methods of obtaining reliable and valid knowledge about empiric experience. Research in the human sciences requires multiple processes to generate empiric knowledge and theory. Empiric knowledge gained from research is considered to be repeatable and valid in its conceptions of reality within given limits. Although research is sometimes used to mean a product, as in the phrase "this is my research," it refers most frequently to the process rather than the outcome.

Fact

A fact is generally held to be an empirically verifiable object, property, or event, meaning that the phenomenon is experienced and named consistently and similarly by others given a similar context. Facts are useful because they reflect common observation on a broad level. If one person observes that it is raining and others agree, the statement "it is raining" is accepted as a fact.

Model

A model is a symbolic representation of an empiric experience. The symbolic form of a model may be words, mathematic notations, or physical material, as in a model airplane. One key idea in understanding models is that they are not the real thing but are an attempt to objectify the concept they represent. A model of any object, property, or event replicates reality with various degrees of precision.

A physical model of some property, event, or object is often useful. The properties and events of the physical and biological world are often modeled to provide a basic understanding of their function. An example is a planetarium, which models the movement of stars and planets in the universe. Modeling human characteristics is difficult, and, when human objects, properties, and events are modeled, the model is less precise because of the complex nature of human characteristics.

It is also possible to model highly abstract concepts. These models consist of such things as words, numbers, letters, or geometric forms. The diagram of the processes for theory development used in this book is an example of a model. Models expressed in language are often called conceptual models, although in one sense all models are conceptual (representative of an idea). Terms sometimes used interchangeably are *conceptual model, conceptual framework, theoretical model,* and *theoretical framework.* For us, conceptual and theoretic models can be presented as a part of theory, can coexist with theory, or can be constructed to show links between related theories.

Paradigm

The term *paradigm* implies a world view or ideology, a medium within which the theory, knowledge, and processes for knowing find meaning and coherence and are expressed. A paradigm implies standards or criteria for assigning value or worth to both the processes and products of a discipline, as well as for the methods of knowledge development within a discipline. All of the components of a paradigm are compatible with one another, but wide variation can exist within its structure.

CONCLUSION

In this chapter, the difficulty of defining concepts was addressed; four definitions of theory were comparatively analyzed, and a new definition was proposed for nursing theory. Definitions of theory-related terms were also discussed, since a full understanding of theory is facilitated by knowledge of its definitions in various contexts. Having established our definition of theory, we will examine the processes for generating and developing theory in Chapter 5.

REFERENCES

Dickoff J and James P: A theory of theories: a position paper, *Nurs Res* 17(3):197–203, 1968.
Dickoff J, James P, and Wiedenbach E: Theory in a practice discipline. Part I: Practice-oriented theory, *Nurs Res* 17(5):415–35, 1968.
Ellis R: Characteristics of significant theories, *Nurs Res* 17(3):217–22, 1968.
Glaser B and Strauss A: The discovery of grounded theory, Chicago, 1967, Aldine Publishing Co.
Jacox A: Theory construction in nursing: an overview, *Nurs Res* 23(1):4–13, 1974.
Kaplan A: The conduct of inquiry, New York, 1964, Thomas Y. Crowell Co, Inc.
Levine ME: The four conservation principles of nursing, *Nurs Forum* 6(1):45–59, 1967.
McKay RP: Theories, models, and systems for nursing, *Nurs Res* 18(5):393–99, 1969.
Rogers ME: An introduction to the theoretical basis of nursing, Philadelphia, 1970, FA Davis Co.
Watson J: Nursing: human science and human care, Norwalk, 1985, Appleton-Century-Crofts.

5

Development of nursing theory

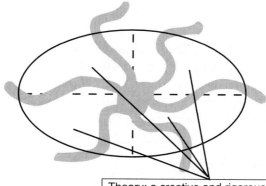

Theory: a creative and rigorous
structuring of ideas that project
a tentative, purposeful, and
systematic view of phenomena.
Chinn and Kramer

There are four processes for creating empiric theory.
These processes are (1) creating conceptual meaning,
(2) structuring and contextualizing theory,
(3) generating and testing theoretic relationships,
and (4) deliberately applying the theory. When all
of these processes occur, theory with practice value evolves.

focus on how concepts are derived

This chapter presents a description of each of the four processes of theory development. Theory can be developed using any of the processes as a starting point.

CREATING CONCEPTUAL MEANING

Creating conceptual meaning provides a foundation for developing theory. Although creating conceptual meaning is a logical starting point for theory development, it does not necessarily have to be accomplished first. It is a process that can be done by the beginning and the advanced scholar and by the novice and expert practitioner (see Chapter 9). As the term for this process implies, we believe that conceptual meaning is something that is created. It does not exist as an "out there" reality, but it is deliberately formed from experience. Although this process is critical to all theory development, it is often overlooked as a component of the process (Norris, 1982). Most theorists provide definitions of terms used within theory, but forming word definitions is not the same as creating meaning. Conceptual meaning conveys thoughts, feelings, and ideas that reflect the human experience of the concept.

We have defined the term *concept* as a complex mental formulation of experience. By "experience," we mean perceptions of the world—objects, other people, visual images, color, movement, sounds, behavior, interactions—the totality of what is perceived. Experience is considered empiric when it can be shared and verified by others using sensory evidence. How the meaning of a concept forms is depicted in Figure 5–1. Three sources of experience interact to form the meaning of the idea: (1) the word or other symbolic label, (2) the thing itself (object, property, or event), and (3) feelings, values, and attitudes associated with the word and with the perception of the thing.

Conceptual meaning is created by considering all three sources of experiences related to the concept—the *word,* the *thing itself,* and the associated *feelings.* The same word may be used to represent more than one phenomenon. For example, the word *cup* may be used to represent several different kinds of objects or ideas. Each use of the word carries with it different perceptions. If the object is a fancy teacup, a very different mental image forms than if the object is the cup into which a golf ball falls on a putting green. The word *love,* a more abstract concept, can be used to describe a feeling toward a parent, child, pet, car, job, friend, or intimate partner.

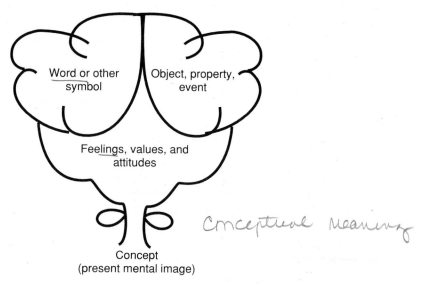

Concept
(present mental image)

Conceptual Meaning

FIGURE 5–1   The formation of concepts.

A single phenomenon can also be represented by several different words. Each word conveys a slightly different meaning, often nuances that related to socially derived value meanings. For example, the words *car, Rolls,* and *hot wheels,* can all refer to one thing—an automobile. Using any of these words to describe the object conveys more about the perspective or value of the person using the word than it does about the object itself. The evolution of words and their multiple meanings are complex.

Conceptual meaning is created, in part, by increasing our awareness of the range of possible uses and meanings of words. Creating conceptual meaning formulates as exactly as possible what is intended so that members of the discipline can follow the reasoning and logic on which a theory is based.

Feelings, values, and attitudes are inner processes that are associated with experiences and words. For example, the word *mother* carries feelings, values, and attitudes that form in human experience with an actual person. Varying experiences with mother (the person) account for a range of feelings that different people associate with the word *mother.* At the same time, human meaning of the concept mother is formed from cultural and societal heritages that all people of a culture share, regardless of individual experiences in early childhood.

Creating conceptual meaning is a theory-building approach that depends on mental processes. This means that mental structures, or ideas, are used to represent experience. What is mentally constructed is expressed in words. This process draws on empiric, esthetic, ethical, and personal knowing in that mental representations using language depend on creativity that comes from the whole of knowing. The process of creating conceptual meaning assumes common yet unique human experiences and shared meaning among people. At the same time, it is a process that assumes that a person's own subjective construction of reality is more accessible than anything else.

The process of creating conceptual meaning brings dimensions of meaning to a conscious, communicable awareness. Because of the limits of language, the process of creating conceptual meaning also makes it possible to identify the limits of understanding meaning. Language limitations for expressing meaning lead to discovery and creativity and form avenues for expanding observable referents (empirics), for increasing self-awareness (personal knowing), for conveying creative dimensions of meaning (esthetic knowing), and for suggesting value (ethical knowing).

The power of language is the power of naming and creating meaning. If a person is told that she is clever, an awareness of self begins to form that may be new to her. At the same time, the word *clever* does not adequately express her rich inner experiences and may not be consistent with her self-knowing. If the word represents a desired value, the description given to her contributes positively to her self-awareness. The process of creating conceptual meaning and naming draws on and contributes to the whole of knowing.

There are various methods for creating conceptual meaning. Berthold (1964) described a method for theoretic and empiric clarification of concepts that was closely linked to the tenets and methods of traditional science. Norris (1982) described several different methods for concept clarification. The methods we suggest here arise from our own experience of concept clarification and are informed by the works of Wilson (1963) and Walker and Avant (1988). They are not a cookbook approach to achieving a final product. They are exercises, mental gymnastics, and techniques that require critical approaches to uncovering subtle elements of meaning that can be embedded in concepts. Theories, which are constructed from clarified concepts, help to unravel hidden or difficult nuances of experience that otherwise might remain hidden from view. Methods for creating conceptual meaning are intended to contribute to theory development by strengthening the conceptual quality of theory.

Creating conceptual meaning produces a tentative definition of the concept and a set of tentative criteria for determining if the concept exists in a particular situation. We use the word *tentative* because both the definition and the criteria can be revised. The term *tentative* does not mean that anything goes or that any definition that suits the author will do. This process is a deliberative, disciplined activity. The person who is creating meaning draws on many information sources, examines many possible dimensions of meaning, and presents ideas so that they can be tested and challenged in the light of purposes for which the concept is being clarified.

Steps

1)

Selecting a concept

An early step in the process of creating conceptual meaning is to select the concept—a word or phrase that communicates the idea you wish to convey. An initial concept may change as meanings evolve. Since experience is not adequately expressed in common language, words may seem quite inadequate at first. You may select a common language word for a concept and eventually assign a specific definition to the word to suit your particular purposes. Or you may borrow a word from another language, combine two or more common words to specify a particular meaning, or make up a phrase or a word. Words that are created to convey a special meaning within a discipline are called technical or professional terms. These words may only have special meaning within disciplines and have no general or common meaning, or, on the other hand, they may be words that are also used in common language.

Selecting a concept is a process that involves a great deal of ambiguity. You will probably not be satisfied with your early choice of terms to express your ideas. Trying out various alternative words becomes part of the process itself. For example, there is no adequate single term for the idea expressed in the phrase "the use of humans as objects." The term *objectification* is close, but it implies some experiences that do not involve the use of humans. The process of working with various terms related to this idea will help to explore various meanings that are possible.

Why?

Clarifying your purpose

To provide a sense of direction, you must know why you are creating conceptual meaning. One purpose is to set boundaries or limits so you don't become hopelessly lost in the process. For example, your purpose might be to work with the concept dependence for a research project. Eventually you need a clear conceptualization of dependence, as well as ideas about how to measure or assess dependence. Another purpose might be to differentiate between two closely related concepts such as sympathy and empathy. In this case, your concern is to create definitions that do this, based on thorough familiarity with meanings that are possible.

Another reason for creating conceptual meaning is to examine the ways in which concepts are used in existing writings. The concept of intuition, for example, frequently appears in nursing literature with diverse meanings. The meanings conveyed reflect different assumptions about the phenomena. As you become aware of these meanings, you can explore the extent to which the meanings are consistent with your own purpose.

Other purposes for creating conceptual meaning include generating research hypotheses, formulating nursing diagnoses, and developing computerized data bases for clinical decision making. Creating conceptual meaning is also a valuable process for learning critical thinking (Kramer, 1993). Whatever your purpose, keeping it as clear as possible can provide a sense of direction when you seem to be hopelessly lost.

Sources of evidence

Once a concept has been selected, the process of creating conceptual meaning proceeds by using multiple sources from which you generate and refine criteria that include indicators for the concept. The sources you choose and the extent to which you use various sources depend on your purposes.

Definitions. One source that provides information about conceptual meaning are definitions and word usages of the concept you are exploring. Existing definitions are often circular and will not give a complete sense of meaning for the concept, but they do help to clarify common usages and ideas associated with the concept. Existing definitions often help to identify core elements about objects, perceptions, or feelings that can be represented by the word. They are also useful to trace the origin of words that give clues to core meaning.

Dictionary definitions provide synonyms and antonyms and convey commonly accepted ways in which words are used. They are not designed to explain the full range of perceptions associated with a word, particularly when the word has a unique use with a discipline or represents a relatively abstract concept.

Existing theories provide a source of definitions that sometimes extend beyond the limits of common linguistic usage. Theoretic definitions and ways in which concepts are used in the context of the theory convey meanings that pertain to the domain of the discipline from which the theory comes.

The term *mother* as defined in the dictionary, for example, refers to the social and biological role of parenting and includes a few characteristics of the role, such as authority and affection. In the context of psychologic theories, the meanings conveyed with respect to the values, roles, functions, and characters of people who are mothers are almost endless and include parenting, physical care, guilt, responsibility, power, and powerlessness.

Cases. Another useful approach to creating conceptual meaning is constructing cases that represent the experience you are exploring. This involves presenting an object or instance of the experience or constructing a scenario that illustrates the experience. From these cases, you can identify and reflect on criteria for the concept.

Model cases.   One type of case is a model case. In constructing a model case, you describe or present an instance of an experience so that "If this is not X, then nothing is." This represents the concept to the best of your present understanding. For concrete concepts such as cup, a model case is relatively easy. An ordinary teacup, for example, can be presented for everyone to see and hold. The people who examine the object can then verify "If this is not a cup, then nothing is." To demonstrate the concept red (a property), a model case is more difficult. You can physically present to the group something that you perceive as red in color and find out if they agree that this is what red is.

When you deal with highly abstract concepts, the task of constructing model cases is more difficult. Usually, model cases of abstract concepts involve experiences and circumstances that are described in words. Model cases may be created from your own experience, or you may find cases in the literature that have been constructed or described by others. For a concept such as mothering, your model case might begin with an event: an infant cries, and an adult picks up the infant. The event is a start, but your observers might object, saying that this description represents only the physical act of picking something up and is not necessarily mothering. Your model case develops until there is enough substance so that people respond to the case by forming a mental image of mothering. As you build on the scenario of an adult picking up an infant to represent mothering, you could include various circumstances, behaviors, motives, attitudes, and feelings that surround the act of picking up the infant. You paint a picture, or tell a story, so that people can confirm that this indeed is mothering. As this and other model cases are created, you can compare various meanings in the experience and define commonalities and differences.

It is often useful to alternatively include and exclude various features of model cases in order to reflect on how central each feature is to the meaning you are creating. For example, in the model case of mothering, the adult might initially be portrayed to be female. Later, you might portray a male adult in the same case. In the absence of any evidence one way or the other, you might tentatively decide that the idea of mothering you are creating will be deliberately limited to instances involving female adults. Since your decision is tentative, you can change your construction for another purpose or circumstance. You can acknowledge the fact that some males mother, but for your purpose your idea deliberately includes the characteristic of female adults.

While you are working with model cases, pose the question What is it that makes this an instance of this concept? The responses to this question form the basis for a tentative list of criteria. In early stages, the criteria may be quite detailed and may be the essential characteristics associated with the concept, given the meanings you deliberately decide to include. The criteria are designed to make it possible to recognize the concept when it occurs and to differentiate this concept from other related concepts. For example, in the case of mothering, you would want to be able to recognize mothering when it happens and distinguish mothering from such related phenomena as caring, nurturing, or helping.

Impressions regarding the criteria begin to form as you design model cases. As you work with various possible features of the model cases, you begin to form ideas about which features are essential and why, as well as their qualitative features. These ideas become the criteria for the concept. Sometimes model cases are presented after clarification is complete. In these instances, the model case is similar to a definitional form for the concept. Here, we use model cases as a way to create, not to represent, meaning.

Contrary cases.   Contrary cases are those that are certainly *not* an instance of the concept. These may be similar in some respects, but they represent something that most observers would recognize easily as what you are *not* talking about. For concrete concepts, contrary cases are relatively easy. A saucer or a spoon can be presented, and most observers in Western cultures would agree that these things are not cups. A spoon may hold liquids that people sip from, but it would not be a cup. A saucer that a cup sits on would also clearly not be a cup. A contrary case for the color red might be the color green. For the concept of restlessness, calmness could be presented as a contrary case.

As you consider contrary cases, ask What makes this instance different from the concept that was selected? By comparing the differences between model and contrary cases, you will begin to revise the model cases. In turn, you can also revise, add to, or delete from the tentative list of criteria that are emerging. For example, one of the traits that distinguishes a cup from a saucer or a spoon is the shape of the cup. You might already discern that this is an essential feature by looking only at the cup. But, when you see the spoon and saucer, the shape stands out in sharp contrast, and your description of essential features of the shape of the cup can be more complete and precise. As you compare the objects, you may also decide that the volume of liquid that a cup holds is an important distinguishing characteristic. Later, when you consider miniature teacups as cases, you might decide that volume is not an essential quality, especially if your other criteria are sufficient to distinguish which objects can be called a cup for your purpose.

Sometimes in creating narrative contrary cases, the tendency is to simply reverse the situation depicted in the model case. Usually, this does not add significant new information to the analysis. If you are having difficulty constructing a negative case, ask someone else to suggest a contrary case or something that is definitely *not* what you are trying to describe. Sometimes you can locate a contrary case in the literature. Contrary cases that contribute to the analysis often reveal important aspects of the model case that are hidden in assumptions that you may be making about the concept.

Related cases. Related cases are instances that represent a different but similar concept. A different word is generally used to label these instances, but the experience has several features in common with the one you have selected for study. When you consider related cases, your ideas become much clearer about the meanings that are central to the concept you are exploring.

In the case of a cup, you might consider a drinking glass. For the concept of red, you might consider a red-orange hue and a magenta. For the concept of mothering, you could design a case of tending that would be similar to the model case. You might make a child-care worker the adult person or substitute an elderly person for the infant. Again, you consider differences and similarities between the model and related cases and revise the tentative criteria to reflect your new insights.

Borderline cases. A borderline case is an instance of metaphoric or pseudo-applications of the word. The same word is generally used for these instances, but the context of use is usually quite different from the one you have selected for study. Poetry and lyrics to music provide rich sources of metaphoric uses of words. In the evolution of language, the metaphoric meanings of words carry powerful messages that often persist as new usages emerge and thus illuminate core meaning. The metaphoric meanings for the concept of red are an excellent example. Red as a word and as a color has become a symbol for communism. The metaphoric messages in this usage symbolize human experiences of blood, violence, passion, and loss. To give a "cup of cheer" is an exemplary borderline usage of the term *cup*. This highlights the feature of cups as capable of holding something.

For the concept of mothering, a borderline case could be a computer "mother board." You might use this case to help clarify features of the concept of mother that can be seen as foundational to the concept, such as the central importance of mother in defining the scope of relationships, or structuring the energy of all relationships in the system. Ask what happens to your meaning if you perceive of mothering as a process that structures and directs the nature of relationships in a system.

You will probably invent other varieties of cases in the process of creating conceptual meaning. How cases are classified is not critical. Their important function is to assist you in discerning the full range of possible meaning so that you can design a meaning that is useful for your purpose.

Visual images.   Visual images that already exist, such as photographs, cartoons, calendars, paintings, and drawings, are useful sources in creating conceptual meaning. You might deliberately create images that represent the concept being clarified rather than use existing sources. The images chosen may be explicitly labeled or named with the concept of interest, or they may be judged to reasonably represent it. If you can find images that others have explicitly labeled as an instance of the concept, such as a picture that the artist labels "sorrow," the artist's link of the visual image and the concept provides further validation of the meaning of the concept and helps to minimize any bias inherent in your own views of meaning for concept.

Whether you personally create and examine an image or ask others to create images, the idea is to compare them for similarities and differences. Advertisements and photographs documenting the concept depression, for example, provide information about conceptual meaning. Often, visual imagery will highlight some aspect of the concept that is significant. On other occasions, visual imagery may raise questions about the essential nature of the phenomena that are important to refining criteria. Visual images that represent concepts very well also highlight difficulties in expressing meaning linguistically. A photograph may express the concept of dignity, yet the essence of dignity expressed by the photo is impossible to describe.

Popular and classical literature.   A variety of literature resources can provide information about conceptual meaning. Whereas cases often evolve from your personal experience, the literature reflects meanings arising from the culture. Classical prose and poetry are often rich sources of meaning for concepts used in nursing. For example, images of love and longing may be found in the poetic works of Emily Dickinson. Louisa May Alcott's classic story, *Little Women,* provides information about the nature of intimacy and caring. The popular current literature is also a source of valuable data about conceptual meaning. Popular self-help books on such topics as stress management and codependency can often clarify commonly understood conceptual meanings. Fairy tales, myths, fables, and stories provide relevant insights, depending on the concept you are exploring. Usages for words that are expressed in popular jargon and cartoons may highlight borderline meaning. For example, when a 5-year-old jumps up and down and exclaims "I'm so *anxious* for my birthday to be here!" the meaning of "anxious" is not the same meaning for anxiety that concerns nurses. What the child's usage conveys is the physical agitation that accompanies the experience of anxiety within the context of nursing practice.

Music and poetry.   The imagery of music or poetry may be useful in concept clarification. Music or poetry can be chosen by seeking out lyrics or titles that name the concept under consideration. Or, the music itself, or the metaphoric images in the title or lyrics, may reasonably suggest the concept. Music and poetry can effectively convey meanings through rhythm, tones, lyrical or linguistic forms and metaphors, or musical moods that reflect experiences in life events with which nurses deal. For example, the Shaker folk tune "Simple Gifts" suggests criteria for concepts of authenticity, genuineness, centeredness, and community. The tune itself conveys a sense of inner happiness and peace; the lyrics reflect relationships between inner peace and the ability to build strong relationships. The popular song "Don't Fence Me In" conveys through the musical mood, rhythm, and lyrics what it feels like to be confined emotionally and projects the yearning to be free.

Professional literature.   Meanings for concepts can be explored from within the context of professional literature. This literature often provides meanings that are pertinent to the practice of nursing. For example, philosophers, as well as nurses, have written about the concept of presence as a way of being with another. Both are valuable sources for exploring meanings. When the literature of other disciplines is considered, meanings may not clearly apply to nursing, but meaning found across disciplines contributes to concept clarification.

People.   Peers, coworkers, hospitalized persons, and professional workers who are not nurses can provide valuable information about the meaning of a concept. It may be useful to seek the opinions of others about the meaning a concept has, particularly if your direct experience with the concept is limited. Nurses who work with the concept daily may be able to shed light on nuances of meaning that will markedly affect how meaning is integrated into theory. For example, a nurse who works with people whose lung function is severely compromised might observe that anxiety, although usually characterized by increased activity, evokes a different reaction. Rather than random activity, it may be accompanied by a deliberate quieting of behavior to conserve energy.

The sources that can be used in creating conceptual meaning are potentially inexhaustible. Undoubtedly you will think of others who are useful to you as you work on clarifying concepts. What sources to use and how to use them unfold as you engage in the process of exploring and creating conceptual meaning.

Exploring contexts and values

Social contexts within which experience and the values that grow out of experience occur from important cultural meanings that influence mental representations of that experience. Consider, for example, the concept of judgment if you are a student taking an examination, a realtor assessing a home for sale, a person scoring a gymnastics meet, or a magistrate preparing to levy a sentence. When you explore the various meanings acquired by virtue of the context, you will probably become aware of meanings you had not previously considered.

One way to imagine various contexts is to place your model cases in different contexts and ask What next? You mentally imagine the practical outcomes of your conceptual meaning in its context. For example, if you place your model case of the color red in the context of a magazine advertisement, what symbolic meaning is conveyed? What advertising results does the advertiser intend? If the color red is placed in the context of traffic signs and symbols, what meaning does the color now convey? What behavioral responses do you now expect? As you consider various possible combinations of context, you will clarify how meanings are influenced by the context.

Values are also revealed by placing the concept in a subtly differing context. The concept of mothering has a relatively positive connotation for most people. Most people agree that humans need "good" mothering to grow and develop adequately. But people differ widely in what they consider to be "good" mothering; these differences often have to do with the cultural context. For example, there would probably be considerable disagreement as to whether what happens in a schoolroom, in a hospital, or in counseling is mothering. What is considered mothering reflects deeply embedded cultural values. When you consider your model case placed in several different social contexts, you create an avenue for perceiving important values and make deliberate choices concerning them.

Formulating criteria

Criteria for the concept emerge gradually and continuously as you consider definitions, various cases, other sources, and varying contexts and values. Criteria are always tentative, but they provide guidelines for recognizing the experience you want to represent and for differentiating it from other similar instances.

As you develop the criteria, you will naturally refine them so that they reflect the meaning you intend. Criteria should express both qualitative and quantitative aspects of meaning and should suggest a definition of the word. Since criteria are more complex than a limited word definition, they amplify this meaning and suggest direction for the processes of developing theory.

To illustrate the function of criteria for a concept, consider how you might convey the idea of one U.S. dollar in coins to a person who is not familiar with American money. One way is to present all possible combinations of coins to the individual, who then memorizes the combinations in order to consistently collect the right coins together to yield an equivalent of $1. Another approach is to provide guidelines to assist the individual to recognize and compose the various combinations independently. A model case might be presented using three quarters, one dime, two nickels, and five pennies.

Realizing many other combinations are possible, criteria are created from the model case to cover all other possible combinations. The model case is chosen deliberately to include all the types of coins available, so that in examining the case, several characteristics of all possibilities emerge. One feature is that the units of the various coins used add up to an equivalent of 100 pennies—the smallest possible coin value. However, this criterion alone may not be sufficient for someone who is not familiar with the monetary system being used; thus, other criteria are created to ensure that all other possible combinations are recognized. You might consider the weight of the possible coin combinations, the colors of the coins, their metallic makeup, or the exchange value of each coin. All of these features may be used, but criteria should convey, as simply as possible, the information needed by a novice to collect one U.S. dollar in coins. The fact is that any color combination or any number of coins up to 100 may be used as criteria. Metallic content of the coins might serve as an adequate criterion and may even be the most precise of all possible criteria. But if your purpose is to assist a person from another country to understand how to make a dollar out of change, you would not select the metallic content as a criterion because it is impractical for that purpose.

For concrete objects, criteria may be relatively simple. For the concept of cup, examples of criteria may be as follows:

1. The object is cylindrical or conical in shape, with one closed and one open end.
2. The object is capable of containing physical matter.
3. The height is between 3 and 7 inches, and the widest diameter is 3 to 4 inches.
4. When the object contains liquid, it must be capable of safely holding hot liquids.

Notice that this set of criteria is phrased so that a styrofoam cup or golfing green cup can be included. This choice is guided by the purpose. If you needed to make sure that the golfing green cup was not included as a cup, you might revise the criteria to include "the object is capable of being held in the hand, regardless of what it contains." This criterion places a limit on the volume and weight of the cup and implies that it must be a portable object.

Developing criteria for more abstract concepts is a more complex process, and the criteria are often more abstract. Criteria for the concept of mothering might be:

1. Visual contact must be observed to be directed from the mothering person to the person who receives mothering.
2. The person who receives mothering must be physically touched by the mothering person.

3. Some positive feeling must be experienced by the mothering person and by the person who receives mothering.
4. There must be a reciprocal interaction between the two people.
5. Vocalization by the mothering person must occur.

These criteria do not limit the mothering person by gender, age, or species. The mother could be an elderly, male person. Nor do the criteria specify that the person who receives mothering is an infant. If the purpose of applying the criteria is to distinguish between instances of mothering and fathering, these criteria would need to be revised to at least specify gender. If the purpose were to differentiate between mothering and neglect, they might be adequate.

A frequent question that arises in the course of creating conceptual meaning is How do I know that the meaning I have created is adequate? You can examine your conceptual meaning for adequacy in relation to the processes used for creating meaning, as well as the conceptual meaning itself that you have created. Fuller (1991) suggests examining the process and the product of conceptualization in terms of both validity and reliability. A conceptualization is valid if it is based on multiple examples that are fully representative of the range of meanings for the concept, if you used multiple interpretive stages during the clarification process, and if the essential structure (or pattern) of the concept can be understood from the criteria. The conceptualization is reliable if the concept can be consistently recognized using the criteria that you have created. The meaning you create is also adequate if it reflects a reasonable and communicable understanding that is useful for your purposes. If your aims reflect valued nursing goals, if you have been careful in choosing and using resources, and if you understand why you have made the choices you have, you will have created an adequate and useful meaning. Additional processes for theory development will provide a check on conceptual meaning and will help refine and illuminate whether the meaning created is valuable.

Conceptual meaning and problems of theoretic development

Problems associated with conceptual meaning often underlie other problems involved in developing theory. A major challenge with respect to generating and testing theoretic relationships is the selection of empiric indicators for a concept. When research reports give conflicting results, the differences are sometimes tied to the use of different definitions and empiric indicators for the concept. If you explore the conceptual meanings within research reports, you can often clarify the extent to which differing conceptual meanings account for the differing research findings. As you carry out the processes for creating conceptual meaning, you will be able to suggest a full range of possible empiric indicators for a concept. You will also be able to identify the limits of empiric approaches in specifying indicators for a phenomenon.

Consider, for example, the concept of mothering and the sample criteria we gave in the previous section. These criteria include characteristics that can be observed empirically. They are reciprocal interaction, visualization, touch, and vocalization. The criterion that states that "some positive feeling must be experienced by the mothering person and by the person who receives mothering" might be one of the most important distinguishing features of your intended meaning for mothering, but it does not easily lend itself to objective observation. It can be assessed indirectly by asking mothers to describe their feelings.

Conceptual meaning is fundamental if you must distinguish one concept from another closely related one. This is often the case when you are generating and testing relationships or structuring and contextualizing theory. The processes of creating conceptual meaning make it possible to propose differentiating features that guide research and theory–structuring activities. Consider the concepts of tending and mothering. Individuals tend to the needs of others in many different contexts, and mothers tend children. A question to be resolved might be Is there a particular kind of tending that occurs with mothering? You can examine a related case of a sitter tending children to determine if any characteristic of tending is within your idea of mothering. As you explore various differentiating features of the central concept, your ideas will become clearer, and the structure of your theory or research study will improve. Concept clarification helps to make decisions about the qualitative dimensions of criteria, such as whether they always need to be evident or if they may be expressed with different intensities. For example, you may decide that, for the concept of mothering, the expression of positive feeling *must* be present, but the degree to which it occurs may vary.

In creating conceptual meaning, the challenge is to evolve a useful and adequate meaning from among a range of possibilities. Although the processes for creating conceptual meaning are in and of themselves useful, you move toward refinements of your meaning that are useful for the full range of research, practice, and theory development when you also project how you mean it to be applied in other activities of theory development.

STRUCTURING AND CONTEXTUALIZING THEORY

Structuring and contextualizing theory involves forming systematic linkages between and among concepts, resulting in a formal theoretic structure. There are many approaches that can be used (Dubin, 1978; Newman, 1979; Reynolds, 1971; Walker and Avant, 1988). The choice of a particular approach depends on your purposes for developing theory, what you already know or assume to be true, and your underlying philosophic ideas about the nature of nursing knowledge. If you begin with an entirely new idea about something and with very little reported about it in the existing literature, the form of the theory that you construct may be a categorization of the concepts into a relational taxonomy that essentially describes your ideas. If you begin with an idea that builds on other theorists' descriptions, you might develop a theoretic structure that provides explanations of complex interrelationships between concepts. If you are structuring theory as an outcome of grounded research, the interrelationships between data clusters guide the structure you create for the theory.

Approaches to structuring and contextualizing theory include

- *Identifying and defining the concepts.* Identifying and defining concepts specify the ideas on which the theoretic structure is built. Definitions can evolve from the processes of creating conceptual meaning, borrowed from other theories, or formulated from multiple other sources. They should identify as clearly and concisely as possible the theoretic meaning of important concepts within the theory.
- *Identifying assumptions.* Identifying assumptions clarifies the basic underlying truths from which and within which theoretic reasoning proceeds.
- *Clarifying the context within which the theory is placed.* Contextual placement describes the circumstances within which the theoretic relationships are expected to be empirically relevant. Clear statements regarding context are particularly important if the theory is to be applied in practice.
- *Designing relationship statements.* Designing theoretic statements describes the projected and evolving relationships between and among the concepts of the theory. These statements, taken as a whole, provide the substance and the form of the theory.

Identifying and defining concepts

Structuring theory requires that you identify the concepts that will form the basic fabric of theory. The concepts can come from life experiences, clinical practice, basic or applied research, knowledge of the literature, and from the formal processes of creating conceptual meaning. Often, theory emerges because of a conviction that existing knowledge and theories are not adequate to represent an experience.

Some concepts are better suited for theory development than others. Concepts that are extremely abstract carry broad meanings and refer to a wide range of experience. These are usually not suitable as a beginning point for theory development. Concepts such as social structure, politics, or love, for example, refer to such a broad range of experience that defining them within the limits of empiric inquiry is extremely difficult. Such concepts, however, can be useful in considering the context within which the theory is placed. If concepts are extremely narrow and concrete, they refer to only a narrow range of experiences, and the level of abstraction may not be sufficient for theoretic purposes. For example, concepts such as toothache, post-surgical pain, or backache apply to relatively few instances of pain. Pain may be a more suitable concept from which to develop theory.

As the concepts are specified or begin to form, early ideas about the structure of their relationships begin to emerge. There are usually one or two primary or central concepts around which the theoretic relationships build. Thinking about possible relationships helps to clarify what concepts the theory needs to include. Previous research, existing theories, philosophies, and personal experience provide a background for forming theoretic relationships. Initially, you might simply note concepts that you think are related on the basis of your experience, what you find in the literature, or ongoing research.

An assumption that is inherent in most empiric theory is the concept of linear time. If your emerging theory is to be predictive, time may influence the type and substance of the concepts required for the theory. Antecedent, coincident or intervening, and consequent concepts imply prediction within a linear time frame. Antecedent concepts are those experiences that you identify as coming before other concepts. Coincident concepts are those that co-exist in time. Intervening concepts are also coincident and have a particular influence on relationships among concepts that are specified in the theory. Consequent concepts are those that follow another.

Some theories place antecedents in a causal relationship with those that follow. Other theories rest on a philosophic view that rejects the idea of causation. Instead, the ideas of influence or affect are used to explain relationships over time. If a primary concept within your developing theory is stress, you might propose that previous childhood experiences cause the stress experience, or you might consider childhood experience as an antecedent that influences the stress experience.

Consequents can also imply causation. For example, once a person experiences stress, consequents of that experience can be thought of as resulting from the stress. Changes in mental functioning, in sleep and rest patterns, and in relationships with other people might be theoretic concepts structured to reflect phenomena caused by the stress.

Intervening concepts can be used to shift from a view of causation to one of influence. Intervening concepts are those that influence the relationships between antecedent experiences, the event itself, and its consequents. For example, the central concept of stress might be viewed as being influenced by the antecedent experiences of childhood, and sleep patterns might be viewed as an intervening variable that influences the relationship between the childhood experience and present stress.

As initial ideas are formed concerning relationships between concepts, the concepts themselves become clearer. Some concepts might be grouped together and assigned more abstract terms to compose a new concept. This occurs especially when theory is structured using inductive theory development processes such as grounded theory. For example, you might begin to see that time of day and season of year could be grouped to become components of the more abstract concept of biologic rhythms.

As the concepts of the theory are identified and conceptualized, theoretic definitions emerge. Theoretic definitions form the basis for and reflect empiric indicators and operational definitions for concepts that are needed for research and convey the general meaning of the concept. Operational definitions are different from theoretic definitions in that they indicate as exactly as possible how the concept is to be assessed in a specific study (see pp. 98–99). For example, a theoretic definition for the concept of mothering might read:

> **mothering**   An interaction between a human adult and child that conveys reciprocal feelings of attachment. The interaction is behaviorally expressed by reciprocal visual contact, touching, and vocalization.

This theoretic definition gives a general idea of empiric indicators for the concept, which in turn imply operational definitions. The first part of the definition provides a general meaning for the term. The second part suggests behaviors associated with the concept that can be assessed.

Notice that the theoretic definition is consistent with tentative criteria for the concept mothering (see p. 89), but the definition serves a different purpose from the criteria. The criteria are specific and useful as a foundation for construction of theory and for empiric study of the concept. The theoretic definition summarizes the insights that are formed in creating conceptual meaning and concisely conveys the essential meaning of the concept.

Identifying assumptions as part of theory

Assumptions are underlying givens that are presumed to be true. They are not intended to be empirically tested for soundness, but they can be challenged philosophically and may be investigated empirically. Philosophic assumptions form the philosophic grounding for a theory; if they are challenged, the substance of the entire theory is also challenged on philosophic grounds. Nonphilosophic assumptions (that is, assumptions that could be empirically investigated but aren't within the context of the theory) also affect the value of the entire theory. Stated assumptions are easy to recognize, but many assumptions are implied, or not stated, and are difficult to recognize. An example of an underlying assumption that is usually not stated is Human beings are complex. For theories that involve human experience, this statement can be taken as reasonably true. However, many commonly accepted truths about human existence gain new significance within a theoretic context, and they need to be stated even if they seem self-evident. For example, if a theory were to include the concept death, certain underlying assumptions about the nature of life and death would influence the essential ideas of the theory, and these need to be stated. A theory that is based on the view of death as a transition to another form of life will be very different from a theory that views death as the end of life.

Rogers (1970) made her assumption explicit that human beings are unified wholes possessing their own integrity and manifesting characteristics that are more than and different from the sum of their parts. On the surface, this seems to be a perfectly reasonable and sensible statement, but it is significant because it is an assumption that is not common to all nursing theory. As an assumption, it does not require empiric evidence, but it is fundamental to the relationship statements she proposed. It is the relationships, not the assumptions, that are empirically tested.

Assumptions influence all aspects of structuring and contextualizing theory. If the assumption holism is used as a basis for a theory of mothering, interrelated concepts must be consistent with a holistic view of human experience. Patterns of behavior that reflect the whole would be reflected in the theoretic concepts. These might include patterns of movement and communication. In contrast, if human beings were assumed to be biologic and social organisms, the concepts of a mothering theory might include such concepts as physical responses and cultural mores.

Clarifying the context

Theoretic relationships must be placed within a context if the theory is to be useful for practice. If a theory of mothering is meant to apply only to the interactions of women and children in Western cultures, these limits on the applicability of the theory must be stated. As the theory is extended, it might be found to be useful for other cultures and for other kinds of intimate relationships such as adult-child, adult-adult, or adult-animal interactions. Theory that arises from inductive methods is contextualized as a result of the process itself.

Contexts that are very broad or very narrow limit the applicability of theory. A theory that is cognitively structured as an explanation for many cultures will probably not be useful for any culture. Conversely, a theory that is structured within the context of a single institution (for example, one hospital) will probably not be useful for other settings.

Designing relationship statements

Relationship statements describe, explain, or predict the nature of the interactions between the concepts of the theory. The statements range from those that simply relate two concepts to relatively complex statements that account for interactions among three or more concepts. Theories usually contain several levels of relationship statements, which compose a reasonably complete explanation of how the concepts of the theory interact. The relationships begin to take form as the concepts are identified and emerge, but the process of designing the relationship statements requires specific attention to the substance, direction, strength, and quality of interactions between concepts.

Consider a relationship statement that might be formulated using the concept of mothering. A theorist might propose that, as an adult's visual contact with an infant increases, the infant's visual contact with the adult will also increase. This relationship statement speculates that one event (increased adult visual contact) precedes a second event (increased infant visual contact). This relationship also describes a substantive interaction (visual contact) as a component of mothering. It implies direction (an increase) as part of the interaction.

A more complex relational statement addresses further dimensions of quality, contexts, and circumstances that are proposed. Such a statement might take the form:

Under the conditions of C1 . . . Cn, if X occurs, then Y will occur.

Or, to use the illustration involving the concept of mothering:

When an adult mothering figure and
an infant are in close proximity (C1),

and

when the adult has a negative feeling toward the infant (C2),

and

when the frequency of physical contact is limited (C3),

then,

if the adult's frequency of visual contact decreases,
the infant's frequency of visual contact will also decrease.

A relationship may also be designed to introduce new concepts to the potential theory. Initially, such a relationship might read:

If the infant's frequency of visual contact is not sufficient to satisfy the mother, the adult's frequency of visual contact will increase in a conscious effort to engage the infant in interaction.

This introduces the concept of awareness and a subjectively understood value, not objectively identifiable as positive or negative, for the concept visual contact. That alternate value is "sufficient to satisfy," which is not empirically observable. As the theory is developed further, possible empiric indicators for satisfaction might be created. Or this dimension of the theory might be viewed as something beyond the realm of empirics. In this way, the theory not only stimulates the creation of new empiric knowledge but also opens possibilities for exploring and integrating other ways of knowing. Although empiric theory is primarily designed to propose and create empiric relationships, it can also contain concepts and relationships that integrate ethical, esthetic, and personal knowing.

GENERATING AND TESTING THEORETIC RELATIONSHIPS

Generating and testing theoretic relationships involve a focus on the correspondence of the ideas of the theory with accessible experience (Dubin, 1978; Newman, 1979; Reynolds, 1971; Glaser and Strauss, 1967). Since empiric theories are abstractions of what can be observed in experience, a translation is made from the theoretic to the empiric (deductive approach) and from the empiric to the theoretic (inductive approach). A theory cannot be proven, but it is possible to show empiric support for a theory. If the evidence does not support or create theoretic relationships, the ideas of the theory cannot be sustained as theory. Alternative theoretic explanations are then considered, based on the empiric evidence.

The activity of generating and testing theoretic relationships draws on one or more subcomponents: (1) empirically grounding emerging relationships, (2) naming empiric indicators, and (3) validating relationships through empiric methods.

Empirically grounding emerging relationships

The process of empirically grounding emerging relationships involves connecting experiences with representations of those experiences. When an abstract theoretic relationship is taken as the starting point, the theorist presents empiric evidence that suggests support for the projected relationship. This is usually presented as examples within the narrative explanations of the theory. When this process is taken as the starting point, the theorist selects a social context in which the phenomenon under consideration is likely to be observed and observes the interactions and circumstances of that context. From the observations, the theorist derives relationship statements that are grounded in empiric evidence, a process called grounded theory (Glaser and Strauss, 1967). A variety of inductive approaches can also be used to ground emerging relationships; this gradually evolves into a theoretic structure that can, in turn, form the basis for deducing relationships.

Naming empiric indicators

Empiric indicators and operational definitions are used to represent concepts as variables in empiric research and are empirically formed for concepts arising from inductive approaches. Formally structured theory can propose empiric indicators, but, until these are put into operation in research, they remain speculative. Using the ideas in actual research makes it possible to refine the ideas of the theory.

Consider the following abstract relationship statement:

As the adult's eye contact increases, the infant's eye contact will increase.

A research project is designed to obtain empiric evidence concerning the use of eye contact as an empiric indicator of mothering. Details such as length of gaze and frequency of eye contact are specified for the relatively abstract concept of "eye contact." In order to use these indicators, the researcher creates a method for observing and timing the length of gaze and the frequency of eye contact.

Part of the process for identifying empiric indicators, especially when primarily deductive processes are used, is to state operational definitions. Operational definitions specify the standards or criteria to be used in making the observations. For example, an operational definition of the term *gaze* might be "a steady, direct, visual focusing on an object that lasts at least 3 seconds." This definition indicates what gaze is (the empiric indicator for visual contact), characteristics that are to be used in calling a behavior a gaze (direct visual focusing on an object), and a standard time parameter that distinguishes a gaze from other related behaviors such as a glance or a look.

It is more difficult to refine empiric indicators for concepts that are more abstract than the concept eye contact. Many concepts related to nursing (for example, anxiety, body image, or self-esteem) are highly abstract and cannot be directly measured. Tests and tools have been constructed to provide an indirect estimate of traits such as these. The fact that they cannot be measured directly does not mean they are nonexistent or cannot be assessed. The empiric challenge is to refine ideas about and evidence for empiric indicators so that estimates of relationships can be explored. The difficulties inherent in such situations can be compared to trying to describe what a tomato tastes like. Once a person bites a tomato, that person knows how it tastes. The descriptions of that taste are not at all adequate in comparison to the actual taste experience. Descriptions of concepts like anxiety also fall short of the actual human experience. However, if the concept is important for nursing, even a limited study of the experience can be useful.

One approach that can be used to derive empiric measures for abstract nursing concepts is to use multiple empiric indicators to form operational definitions. For example, anxiety might be measured using a self-report tool. The tool can be constructed to include many sensations that are generally indicative of anxiety. The operational definition of the concept anxiety then becomes what is assessed with the use of the tool. Anxiety might also be empirically assessed by observing a person's behavior and the physiologic indicators of adrenocortical function. The operational definitions would include specific ways to measure the behaviors observed and the specific range of laboratory test results associated with anxiety. All of these empiric indicators are possible. If they are used together in situations in which anxiety is likely to occur, the study will provide substantive evidence about the usefulness of each measure as an empiric indicator.

When inductive research processes form the basis for refining empiric indicators, the indicators are directly or indirectly observed and are used to form concepts. Determining empiric indicators for concepts becomes important when inductively generated empiric concepts are deductively tested and extended into other contexts.

Validating relationships through empiric methods

Generating and testing theoretic relationships also require creating a design that tests designated relationships. Designs may be proposed after theory is structured (deductive) or may generate theory that, because of the design, is considered to be tested.

Systematic research designs that deductively test specific relationships incorporate several features. One is that the design provides a means to ensure that the proposed relationship is actually the one that accounts for the study findings. For example, if a study concludes that a mother's gaze prompts an infant's gaze in return, the researcher needs to consider ways to be sure that it is actually the mother's gaze that accounts for the infant's behavior. Typically, the researcher designs the study so that other factors that could influence the behavior of the infants in the study (for example, sensory experiences such as noise, touch, or visual distractions that might affect the process of visual interaction) are held constant or accounted for. The purpose of deductively testing any relationship statement is to provide empiric evidence that the relationships proposed in the theory are adequate when represented in a specific situation. With each approach to design that is used, the research question or hypothesis is revised to suit the type of design selected. Empiric evidence based on many different approaches to research design provides a basis for judging the adequacy of the theory. If theoretic statements are deductively tested and not supported by empiric evidence, one or more of four possibilities can account for the disparity between the theory and empiric findings:

1. *The meaning of the concepts are not adequately created.* The process of creating conceptual meaning can be used to determine if the definitions and meanings of the concepts under study are clear and if they are well differentiated from other related concepts. If they are not, theoretic revisions can be made, resulting in new approaches to empiric study.
2. *The relationship statement is not adequately structured.* The processes of theory structuring and contextualizing can be used to examine the logic or form of the statements. Given the benefit of the empiric evidence, new insights regarding the form and structure of the theory might emerge. The theorist can revise the theoretic relationship statements on the basis of these insights.
3. *The empiric indicators for the concept are not adequately named.* The empiric evidence might point to new possibilities for empiric indicators or suggest revisions in the existing indicators. This process is particularly important when the empiric indicators represent highly abstract concepts and are constructed out of speculative ideas about how the concepts can be observed empirically.
4. *The operational definitions are inadequate or inconsistent.* Typically, conflicting research results are attributed to faulty operational definitions and the related measurement problems of empiric research. This is a possibility, but accurate measurement depends on adequately conceived concepts, sound theoretic statements, and adequate empiric indicators. If these are all in place, it is then reasonable to consider problems in operationalization.

When inductive methods are used to generate theoretic relationships, the relationships may be considered valid if processes for generating them are carefully done. When relationships are deduced from inductively generated theory, they can be tested. When this occurs, any problems with faulty concepts, relational statements, empiric indicators, and operational definitions will become evident.

DELIBERATELY APPLYING THE THEORY

Deliberately applying the theory draws on research methods to assess how fully the theory can be applied in practice to achieve practice goals. The theoretic relationships are systematically examined in the practice setting, and the results are recorded and assessed to determine how well the theory achieves the desired outcomes. Testing of theoretic relationships may also occur in the clinical setting, but, when this occurs, only a part of the theory is assessed, and the setting is usually altered in order to focus on the theoretic relationship selected for testing. Inductive methods that generate theoretic relationships may evolve from nonpractice settings. The extent to which the theory is useful in practice settings needs to be assessed. Deliberative application of theory shifts the focus from testing and generating relationships to gathering evidence as to how the clinical setting itself is affected by and affects the application of the theory. The question shifts away from the soundness of the theoretic relationships to questions concerning the value of the theory in relation to the goals of nursing.

For example, you might be developing a theory concerning the alleviation of pain. The theory generated from an inductive process and empiric evidence testing the theoretic relationships support the developing theory. Deliberative application involves using the theory in practice to carefully assess and understand the effect of its use on the quality of life, the quality of nursing care, or the processes of health.

Deliberative application of theory has three subcomponents. These are (1) selecting the clinical setting, (2) determining outcome variables for practice, and (3) implementing a method of study.

Selecting the clinical setting

The clinical setting for deliberative application can be any setting where nursing is practiced in which the theoretic relationship can be observed. Some phenomena, such as the experience of powerlessness, alienation, or separation, tend to occur in hospitals or other traditional care settings. Other phenomena, such as decision making, are common to a wide variety of settings, such as homes, workplaces, hospitals, and community centers. The setting is selected in part because the theory under study is perceived to be useful for that setting.

Determining outcomes

The process of determining outcomes moves beyond the domain of the theory to explore how the theory, applied in practice, affects the practice of the nursing. Some of the most general outcomes are those that are reflected in nursing standards of quality of care. The components of process, structure, and outcomes that are defined to represent quality become the variables that are assessed in deliberative application of theory.

Practice goals are sometimes implied or are made explicit as part of the theory. For example, if the relationships of the theory are claimed to evolve from a sense of community among the elderly or if this seems like a reasonable inference, this general practice goal can become the outcome that is assessed in order to estimate the adequacy of the theory to achieve this goal.

Implementing a formal method of study

The methods that are used for this process draw on traditional research methods but shift to include the methods of evaluation and quality-assurance research. In this type of research, the method is designed to provide evidence of the effect of the new approach on the overall well-being of people who receive care, on the technical and professional aspects of the practice of nursing, and on the practice setting. Therefore, the setting itself becomes a major focus for observation.

If, for example, you have a theory of pain alleviation that you wish to apply in practice, you might design a study that would first estimate the quality of nursing care that is provided before the theory is applied in practice. Your assessment could include the perspective of nurses, people receiving nursing care, and the administrators of the agency. After you have this information, you would begin to use the theory in practice and over time continue to observe the same indicators of quality of care. On the basis of your findings, you could make recommendations for practice and for revisions in the conceptualizations of the theory.

CONCLUSION

The interrelated processes for theory development include creating conceptual meaning, structuring and contextualizing theory, generating and testing theoretic relationships, and deliberately applying the theory. Although theory, as we have defined it, can be developed using only conceptual approaches, useful practice theory that assumes research will be generated and theoretic relationships tested. Deliberative application will also occur in practice. Once a theory has been developed, members of the discipline begin to assess the adequacy of the theory, conduct research based on the theory, and explore its applicability in practice. The remaining chapters focus on how a discipline assesses the worth of the theory and makes links between the theory, research, and practice. In Chapter 6, we present the description of theory, a process underlying the assessment and use of existing theory.

REFERENCES

Berthold JS: Theoretical and empirical clarification of concepts, *Adv Nurs Sci* 2(5):406–22, 1964.

Dubin R: Theory building, revised ed, New York, 1978, The Free Press.

Fuller J: A conceptualization of presence as a nursing phenomenon. Unpublished PhD dissertation, 1991, University of Utah.

Glaser B and Strauss A: The discovery of grounded theory, Chicago, 1967, Aldine Publishing Co.

Kramer M: Concept clarification and critical thinking: integrated processes, *J Nurs Educ* 32(9):1–10, 1993.

Newman M: Theory development in nursing, Philadelphia, 1979, FA Davis Co.

Norris CM: Concept clarification in nursing, Rockville, 1982, Aspen Systems Corp.

Reynolds PD: A primer in theory construction, Indianapolis, 1971, The Bobbs-Merrill Company, Inc.

Rogers ME: An introduction to the theoretical basis of nursing, Philadelphia, 1970, FA Davis Co.

Walker LO and Avant KC: Strategies for theory construction in nursing, ed 2, Norwalk, 1988, Appleton & Lange.

Wilson J: Thinking with concepts, London, 1963, Cambridge University Press.

6

Description of nursing theory

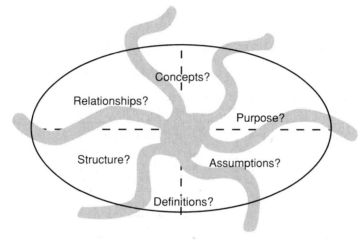

Theory is characterized by certain components that
can be identified, described, and organized by asking,
What is this? As this question is posed, understanding
begins to form. Understanding what a theory is is essential
information for knowing how a theory works or functions.

The definition of theory we use in this text means that theory is characterized by certain theoretical components (see Fig. 4–2). This chapter suggests an approach to describing theory. Processes for critical reflection are the focus of Chapter 7.

COMPONENTS OF THEORY

The definition of theory we use has six descriptive elements. The definition is

> **theory**   A creative and rigorous structuring of ideas that projects a tentative, purposeful, and systematic view of phenomena.

The descriptive components that this definition suggests are

- *Purpose.* Theory is developed for some reason that can be identified. The purpose of a theory may not be stated explicitly, but one should be identifiable.
- *Concepts.* Theories are structured from concepts expressed in language.
- *Definitions.* The concepts of a theory carry identifiable meanings that are conveyed in definitions. Definitions vary in precision and completeness, but conceptual meaning should be identifiable in a theory. The meanings for the concepts created by the theorist give the theory its particular character.
- *Relationships.* Concepts are structured into a systematic form that links each concept with others.
- *Structure.* The relationships between concepts form a whole whereby the ideas of the theory interconnect. The structure makes it possible to follow the reasoning of the theory in its entirety.
- *Assumptions.* Assumptions are the underlying truths that determine the nature of concepts, definitions, purpose, relationships, and structure. Many assumptions are difficult to identify because they are implied rather than explicit. Because they are fundamental, we include assumptions as a describable component of theory, even when they are not stated explicitly.

Describing theory is a process of posing questions about these components and responding to the questions with your own reading or interpretation of the theory. Some elements will seem clear; some will depend on tentative interpretations; some will remain unclear. The process of responding to the descriptive questions for each component make it possible to discern that this *is* a theory and what type of theory it is.

POSING QUESTIONS

What is the purpose of this theory?

The general purpose of the theory is important because it specifies the context and situations in which the theory applies. Purpose can be initially approached by asking, Why is this theory formulated? Information about the theorist's sociopolitical context provides insight about circumstances that influenced the creation of the theory. The theorist's experience, the setting in which the theory was formulated, societal trends, philosophic ideas that gave form to the theorist's view, and experience that motivated the creation of the ideas of the theory can all provide insight as to why it was formulated. The responses to this question provide information that pertains to theoretic purposes.

When approaching the question of purpose, it is important to clarify which purposes are embedded in the theoretic structure and which are reasonable extensions of the theory. For example, consider a theory of mother-infant attachment that includes the following concepts: (1) birth or adoption experience, (2) maternal support systems, (3) degree of bonding, and (4) healthy infant development. Healthy infant development is an example of a clinical outcome, or purpose, that is embedded in the structure of the theory. The purpose, quality of life, would be an extension of the theory, since this concept is not found within the structure of the theory. Purposes that are identifiable within the structure of the theory are usually explicit. Purposes that are reasonable extensions of the theory are important to clarifying the clinical usefulness of the theory, but they are not clearly linked to the central structure of the theory. Purposes outside the context of the theory also suggest directions for further development of the theory.

Some purposes require the practice of nursing in order to be achieved. In these theories, the concepts of the theory include nursing actions and behaviors that contribute to the purpose. Pain alleviation and restored self-care ability are examples of purpose that require the practice of nursing and suggest that nursing actions are part of the theory. Note that these purpose statements have a value orientation: alleviation and restoration. These ideas imply change toward a certain goal, not just change for the sake of change. Value connotations such as these are important to understanding the purpose of the theory.

Some purposes may not require the practice of nursing but are useful for understanding phenomena that occur in the context of nursing practice. These purposes can contribute to achieving practice purposes, or they may not be directly relevant to practice goals. Consider, for example, a theory with a central purpose of explaining variables affecting blood flow velocity in the skin. Clinical practice is not necessary to explain blood flow velocity, but a theory with this purpose might be linked to a theoretic explanation of how blood flow velocity influences the incidence of decubiti or the extent of peripheral neuropathy in people with diabetes. A theory that explains skin blood flow velocity would also help practitioners prevent decubiti and peripheral neuropathy.

Theoretic purposes that do not require direct clinical nursing actions but are of concern to nursing may also involve professional issues in nursing. For example, the purpose of a theory might be to describe features of organizations that empower nurses. This valued and necessary purpose is not directly related to the specific nursing actions used in giving care, but it is certainly useful for changing practice.

Purposes within a theory may be found for individuals or for groups of people. For example, if a theory is developed toward the clinical goal of pain alleviation, the theory can be examined for purposes appropriate for the nurse, the physicians, the person receiving care, and the family. Consider theory developed with a clinical purpose of promoting high-level wellness. The role and outcomes for the nurse might be distinctly different from that implied for the person receiving nursing care. The nurse's purpose might be to design a system that promotes recovery. The purpose for the person receiving care might be to recover and to provide responses indicating how effective the system is in promoting recovery. Taken together, these two purposes might be viewed as creating an interacting recovery process.

One question that often arises is, How are purposes to be separated from the concepts of the theory? Purposes that are part of the matrix of the theory are also concepts of the theory. One approach to identifying which concept is also the central purpose is to describe or to designate the concept toward which theoretic reasoning flows. Ask, What is the end point of this theory? and, When is this theory no longer applicable? Responses to these questions provide clues to purpose and help to clarify the context in which the theory can be used. In Hall's theory (1966), for example, the theory would cease to be valuable when the client was self-actualized, and self-actualization may be deemed the overall purpose. This purpose of self-actualization represents the end point of theoretic reasoning. In the context of Hall's theory, self-actualization is a purpose that requires nursing actions. Outside the context of Hall's theory, self-actualization is a purpose that is shared with other professions. Hall's theory provides a nursing context within which self-actualization becomes meaningful.

Another question about purpose concerns the individual, family, group, and societal dimensions of the theory. Does the purpose of a theory apply to society? To groups? To individuals? An adapted society and an expanded collective consciousness are examples of broad purposes that apply to relatively unbounded groups of people. Purposes such as environmental health or political activism apply to communities that can be linked to a definable group of people. The purpose of quality of life can apply to individuals, families, groups, and communities.

What are the concepts of this theory?

Concepts are identified by searching out words or groups of words that represent objects, properties, or events within the theory. You can begin to describe concepts by listing key ideas and tentatively identifying how they seem to relate to one another. As you begin to discern relationships, your perception of the key concepts of the theory will become clearer. One initial difficulty in identifying concepts is identifying which concepts are integral to the theory and which are part of some supporting narrative. There is no easy way to deal with this. By beginning to identify concepts and deriving interrelationships, decisions can be made about which concepts are central to the theory.

As important theoretic concepts are identified, ask questions about the nature of the concepts and their organization. These questions include, Is there a major concept with subconcepts organized under it? Are there several major concepts with subconcepts organized under them? Are concepts singular entities? Are some concepts singular entities and others organized with subconcepts? What are the relationships and interrelationships between and among concepts? Are some concepts mentioned that do not seem to fit the emerging structure? Once concepts are identified and questions such as these are addressed, the relationships and structure will begin to emerge.

Questions dealing with the numbers of concepts include, How many concepts are there? How many might be termed *major* concepts? How many are *minor* concepts? As you consider the organization and quantity of concepts, address qualitative features of the concepts as well. Questions of quality include, Do the concepts represent abstractions of objects, properties, or events? Is it possible to identify what they represent? Are the concepts more empirically grounded, or are they more abstract? What proportion of the concepts is empirically grounded? What proportion is highly abstract? Are the concepts fairly discrete in meaning, or do several have similar meanings? When similar meanings for concepts exist, ask Do they all seem to express a single idea, or are they different? How? Concepts that are alike may represent one central idea that is fairly clear or several different images. For example, the concepts of rehabilitation, restoration, and recovery, which share common meanings, may appear in the same theory with similar meanings or with different meanings.

When you are addressing the question of a theory's concepts, the concepts within it must be examined carefully for quantity, character, emerging relationships, and structure. The description of concepts is crucial because their quantity and character form understanding of the purpose of the theory, the structure and nature of theoretic relationships, the definitions, and the assumptions.

How are concepts defined?

A definition is any explicit or implicit meaning that is conveyed for a concept. Definitions exist to clarify the nature of the abstraction that the theorist constructs in a way that can be comprehended by others. Definitions suggest how word representations of an idea (concept) are expressed in empiric reality.

It is often difficult to determine from a listing of key words which concepts are basic to the theoretic structure and which comprise definitions and assumptions. Carefully reading the theory and relying on your own judgement should provide this information.

Concepts may be defined explicitly such as in a list of definitions, or they may be explicitly defined in narrative form in the text but not labeled as definitions. It is not always easy to recognize implicit definitions, because they are not labeled and are often inferred from implied meanings.

Since concepts may be defined both explicitly and implicitly, ask the following, How are concepts defined? Explicitly? Implicitly? Both? Are implied definitions consistent with explicit definitions? Can common language meanings be taken as the meaning intended? Would a common language approach lead to differing interpretations of the meanings of the concepts?

Another way to describe definitions is to characterize the extent to which the definitions are general or specific. It is possible for both explicit and implicit meanings to be either general or specific. In assessing how general or specific definitions are, ask, How clearly does the definition suggest an associated empiric experience? Is the definition specific about what a phenomena is, or does it suggest what it is used for? Does it provide possibilities for empiric indicators that represent the phenomenon?

For abstract concepts found in many nursing theories, specific definitions are difficult to formulate. Attempting to create specific meanings of abstract concepts prematurely may interfere with exploring a wide range of possibility that leads to discovery. Definitions that specify general features can conjure very specific mental images of the actual experience. An early definition that is broad and nonspecific encourages the exploration of many possible meanings. General meanings are preferred in broad scope theory or theory that is not likely to be empirically tested. Most definitions have both specific and general features. Ask, How are definitions both specific and general?

Once definitions are identified, ask, Are similar definitions used for different concepts? Are differing definitions used for the same concept? Are some concepts defined differently from common convention? Are definitions expanded as the narrative proceeds? Is it difficult to judge whether definitions are provided at all? Can definitions fit other terms within or outside of the structure of the theory?

What is the nature of relationships?

Relationship statements provide links among and between concepts. The nature of relationships in theory may take several forms. Often relationship statements that are uncovered may be peripheral to the core of the theory.

As concepts are identified, ideas about relationships between them begin to form. Suppose you uncover a relationship statement: "The individual is composed of three dimensions and is an integral part of the environment." This suggests that the individual is related to an environment and that there are three interrelated subcomponents of the individual.

Once a tentative identification of relationships is made, ask, Are there concepts that stand alone, unrelated to others? Are there concepts interrelated with other concepts in several ways and others related in only one or two ways? Are there concepts to which several other concepts relate but that, in turn, are not related to other concepts?

The ways in which the relationships emerge provide clues to the theoretic purposes and the assumptions on which the theory is based. Some concepts may be linked to the theory by assumptions. This may explain why the concept seems to fit within the matrix of the theory, but a theoretic relationship containing the concept is not explicitly stated. The theoretic purpose can be represented by the one-way relationships of several concepts with one specific concept that in turn is not linked to any other concepts (that is, the links end with this specific concept). As links between concepts are identified, you can address the nature or character of relationships. If a relationship is unclear, ask yourself what might be possible relationships and their character; your ideas can provide clues for further development of the theory.

Examine the nature of relationships by asking, Are the relationships basically descriptive, or do they explain? Do they create meaning without explaining? Do they impart understanding? Is there evidence that some relationships are predictive? Relationships within theory that create meaning and impart understanding often link multiple concepts in a loose structure. In other forms of description, concepts are interrelated without elaboration on how and why conceptual relationships are arranged. Concepts that are interrelated to explain often convey how empiric events occur and may provide some detail about how and why concepts interrelate. Prediction implies if-then statements about the occurrence of empiric phenomena. When predictions of human behavior are shown to be valid, they are usually based on explanation.

The statement, "Individuals are composed of three dimensions," is mainly descriptive. It implies that one concept, the individual, is composed of three parts called dimensions. If expanded to "The individual is composed of three dimensions that overlap and share common core areas," the statement becomes more explanatory. It proposes that each dimension has a shared area with another dimension and that there is an area shared by all three. When "interrelated whole" is added, the "how" of the relationship becomes even clearer, because the dimensions must overlap to interrelate the parts of the individual.

Predictions are fairly easy to detect. Sentences that translate into if-then statements are predictive. It is not possible to make an if-then statement out of "The individual is composed of three dimensions," unless it is the implied, "If not three dimensions, then not the individual." The statement, "The individual is an interrelated whole composed of three dimensions that overlap and share common areas," implies that disturbances in one sphere would be reflected in other spheres. This prediction, however, is not explicit.

Suppose the statement read, "Because the individual is an interrelated whole composed of three dimensions that overlap and share common areas, a disturbance in one dimension is reflected in disturbances in other dimensions." This statement is clearly predictive. The distinctions between description, explanation, and prediction are not always clear. Generally, description means that the statement projects *what* something is or the features of its character. Explanation suggests *how* or *why* it is. Prediction projects circumstances that create or alter a phenomenon. Our use of descriptive, explanatory, and predictive in describing the nature of theoretic relationships refers only to the form of the theory. In this context, we do not mean to imply that empiric validation or findings are required to discern whether relationship statements are descriptive, explanatory, or predictive.

What is the structure of the theory?

The structure of theory gives overall form to the conceptual relationships within it. The structure emerges from the relationships of the theory. Consider two concepts within a theory: individual and environment. In one theory, individuals are part of the environment, and in another, individuals are separate from the environment. In both theories, there is an identifiable relationship between individuals and environment; however, the structure of the relationship differs, as symbolically represented in Figure 6–1. Since a relationship between two theoretic concepts can take different structural forms, it is important to describe the nature of both.

Although your responses to questions concerning the relationships of theory usually suggest the form, in some cases they do not. Many theories do not contain a single discernible structure where all concepts fit into a coherent, unified network. There may be several, perhaps competing, structures that cannot be reconciled. Determining the structure of theory will be difficult if the network of relationships is unclear or very complex. Figure 6–2 depicts a sample of four structural forms and the ideas they suggest. Some theories may reflect one or more of these structures, whereas others will not. Sometimes individual concepts within theories may be structured in these forms. Structural forms are powerful devices for shaping our perceptions of reality.

Consider how you might structure the relationship statement, "Individuals are composed of component parts." This only suggests a structure in which parts are perceptible, and any image on Figure 6–2 could represent it except the one that suggests polarity. Suppose each of these structures represents the broad theory of health. The triangular drawing suggests that health is composed of a series of related subconcepts that vary in breadth or simplicity. It also suggests foundational concepts on which other subconcepts are built. The base level might be genetic integrity, followed by organ-system health, and finally health of communities or societies. A theory that deals with how genetic health forms the basis for individual, collective, and societal health might be structured this way.

The overlapping circles depict discrete components that have common areas between and among them. Health might be viewed as having biophysiologic, psychoemotional, and sociocultural aspects. If a person is biologically well but psychoemotionally unwell, the diagram suggests that illness will affect biophysiologic wellness. Psychoemotional ill health could result in biophysiologic consequences. Basically, the overlapping circles illustrate that, although health is composed of separate components, there is sharing between any two components, as well as among all three. The structure as illustrated suggests an equality in importance, overlap, and sharing among the three subunits.

Applying this idea to the horizontal line drawing on the figure shows health represented as a continuum—in a linear relationship with illness. When health is placed on a continuum with illness on the opposite end, health and illness are conceptualized as a continuous variable, and degrees of health and illness are possible. The extremes of a continuum also suggest that health is the absence of illness, and illness is the absence of health. If health is viewed as a concept that is continuous with illness, health and illness can be represented by a continuum. If health and illness are considered as entirely different concepts, they do not fit this structural form. A relationship between gender and society could not be represented on a continuum, for example.

The fourth structural form conveys the idea of differentiation, dividing major concepts into subconcepts. For this structural form, health might be differentiated into its mental and physical aspects. Physical health could be further divided into bodily or anatomic health and functional or physiologic

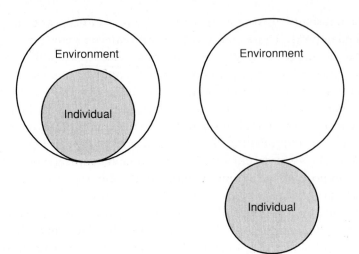

FIGURE 6–1 Alternate structure forms for individual-environment relationships.

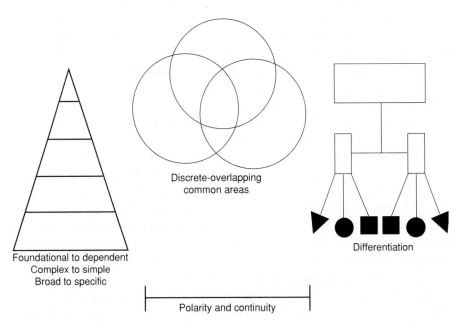

FIGURE 6–2 Structural idea forms.

health, with some comparable division such as emotional and spiritual for mental health. Differentiation can proceed indefinitely. Some concepts lend themselves to differentiation more easily than others. Needs is a concept that can be easily differentiated, whereas the concept of holism cannot.

As you study the examples of structure, note how different concepts fit some structures more easily than others and how some concepts such as holistic health cannot be represented well by any of them. In fact, none of these structures for representing health may make sense for you because they are inconsistent with your personal ideas about the nature of health.

As relationships are explored, the overall theoretic structure and the structure of individual components begin to emerge. To address questions of structure, begin by asking, What are the most central relationships? What is the direction, strength, and quality of relationships? Can I draw a model that shows the structure of the theory? What is the order of appearance of relationships within the narrative? Do relationships appear to move toward or away from the theoretic purpose? Do relationships coalesce concepts or differentiate them? Does the theorist diagram the structure?

Once the structure of the major or central relationships is identified, other aspects of structure can be described. Ask How are other structures united with central or core relationships? Can all relationships be structured? Do the structures take multiple forms? Are competing or partial structures suggested? Does the theorist provide diagrams that illustrate aspects of structure?

Once you have structured the relationships, describe the entire structural form. Notice how the relationships move as the theory unfolds. A theory that defies structuring can sometimes be approached by simply outlining the order in which concepts are presented. Outlining can provide insight about how ideas are organized. Some recognizable structure is essential to theory, because structure flows from relationships.

On what assumptions does the theory build?

Assumptions are those basic givens or accepted truths that are fundamental to theoretic reasoning. In order to uncover assumptions, a central question is, What is the author taking as an accepted truth? This question can be asked once the purposes are determined, the concepts are structured by relational statements, and the definitions are described.

Sometimes the theorist states assumptions explicitly. If so, ask, What are they? What do they assume? Statements explicitly labeled assumptions may not be the same as the assumptions that are basic to the theory. The extent to which explicitly labeled assumptions *are* assumptions and not something else must be examined. It is often difficult to separate assumptions that are implicit or integrated into the narrative of the theory from relationship statements, but they can be identified. As with explicit assumptions, ask, What are the implicit givens? What do they assume?

To further explore your ideas about the assumptions of the theory, ask, What individual, environment, nursing, and health-related assumptions are made? Are assumptions competing or compatible? Are there several assumptions about one phenomena and few about another? Are assumptions made at the outset, between and within relationships, or in relation to the purposes of the theory?

Assumptions may take the form of factual assertions, or they may reflect value positions. Factual assumptions are those knowable or potentially knowable through experience. Value assumptions assert or imply what is right, good, or ought to be. Often an empirically knowable assumption such as, "It is assumed for the purposes of this theory that people want information," contains important underlying value assumptions. The assumption that people want information (which could be empirically verified) may further imply that information is good to have, which cannot be verified empirically. The value assumption that it is good to have information leads to further questions about what sort of information is good. It is important to examine factual assumptions by asking, What value does this factual assumption reflect? It is also important to examine all other components of theory and ask, What does this concept, definition, relationship, structure, or purpose assume?

Once you discern assumptions, the values held by the theorist can be explored by asking, What does the theorist assume to be valuable, good, right, wrong, or worthwhile? Are there value-laden terms and phrases in the definitions of concepts and in the supporting narrative of the theory? Who is assumed to be responsible for the experiences or circumstances of the theoretic reality? Who benefits from the circumstances or experiences of this theory? These questions often give clues to values that form fundamental assumptions. For example, the Freudian theoretic notion of penis envy implies that penises are body parts that are so valued as to be enviable and that people who do not have a penis will experience this value-laden emotion. A useful approach to uncovering hidden values is to imagine possibilities other than that presented in the theory. If these alternate possibilities are plausible, but unconventional, you have uncovered important value assumptions. Imagining the idea of womb envy, which is not a part of Freudian thinking but is a plausible alternate possibility, indicates that you have uncovered an important androcentric assumption from which the theory builds.

The descriptive component of assumptions is often based on ideas taken so much for granted that they are difficult to recognize. An example of such an obvious assumption is that reality is what can be perceived and experienced through the senses. This assumption is fundamental to empirics, but it is not an assumption of other patterns of knowing.

Sometimes it is not possible to accept a theory because it is unusual or unfamiliar. Uneasiness or discomfort with a theory is sometimes a clue to assumptions that are unlike your own beliefs or values. Once assumptions are recognized, the theory containing them can be understood on its own terms.

Forming a complete description

In summary, the five questions for describing theory are

- What is the purpose of this theory? This question addresses why the theory was formulated and reflects the contexts and situations to which the theory can be applied.
- What are the concepts of this theory? This question identifies the ideas that are structured and related within the theory. It questions the qualitative and quantitative dimensions of concepts.
- How are the concepts defined? This question clarifies the meaning for concepts within the theory. It questions how empiric experience is represented by the ideas within the theory.
- What is the nature of relationships? This question addresses how concepts are linked together. It focuses on the various forms relationship statements can take and how they give structure to the theory.
- What is the structure of the theory? This question addresses the overall form of the conceptual interrelationships. It discerns whether the theory contains partial structures or has one basic form.
- On what assumptions does the theory build? This question addresses the basic truths that underlie theoretic reasoning. It questions whether assumptions reflect philosophic values or factual assertions.

A general approach that can be used in describing theory is to read the work and then begin to consider the descriptive questions. The outline shown in the box on pp. 118–119 summarizes the questions that can be asked to form a complete description of theory. All questions are not necessarily answerable for a single theory. As you respond to the questions, concepts will be tentatively identified, and the purpose of the theory will emerge. The definitions will become evident, and you will begin to see relationships. From the nature of the relationships, you will be able to address questions concerning the structure of the theory. Responses to questions concerning assumptions provide a level of awareness of meanings and will help you form understanding of the theory. After an initial description of components, each component can be reexamined and revised.

For any theory, it is not easy to describe the theoretic purpose and assumptions, and the description is usually tentative,but these components can be found. Concepts and their definitions are more readily identifiable, especially

GUIDE FOR THE DESCRIPTION OF THEORY

1. Purpose
- Why is this theory formulated?
- Is there an overall purpose for the theory? A hierarchy of purposes? Separate numerous purposes?
- Is there a purpose for the nurse? The person receiving care? Society? Environment?
- How broad or narrow is the purpose?
- What is the value orientation of the purpose? Positive, negative, neutral?
- Does achieving the theoretic purpose require a nursing context?
- Does/do the purpose/purposes reflect understanding? Creation of meaning? Description, explanation, and prediction of phenomena?
- When would the theory cease to be applicable? What is the "end point?"
- What purpose not explicitly embedded in the matrix of the theory can be identified?

2. Concepts
- Is there one major concept with subconcepts organized under it?
- How many concepts are there?
- How many major ones?
- How many minor ones?
- Can the concepts be ordered, related? Arranged into any configuration? Are there concepts that cannot be interrelated?
- Are concepts broad in scope? Narrow?
- How abstract or empiric are the concepts?
- What is the balance between highly abstract and highly empiric concepts?
- Do concepts represent objects, properties, events? Can you say? Are there concepts that are closely related?

3. Definitions
- Which concepts are defined? Which are not?
- Which concepts are defined explicitly? Which are implied?
- How much meaning needs to be inferred?
- Which concepts are defined specifically? Generally?
- Are there competing definitions for some concepts? Are there similar definitions for different concepts?
- Do any explicitly defined concepts not need definition?
- Are any concepts defined contrary to common convention?

GUIDE FOR THE DESCRIPTION OF THEORY—cont'd

4. Relationships
- What are the major relationships within the theory?
- Which relationships are obvious? Which are implied?
- Do relationships include all concepts? Which are not included?
- Are some concepts included in multiple relationships?
- Is there a hierarchy of relationships? Do relationships create meaning and understanding? Do they do this by describing, explaining? Predicting? What mix of each?
- Are relationships directional? What is their direction? Are they neutral?
- Are there mixed, competing, or incongruous relationships?
- Are relationships illustrated?

5. Structure
- How are overall and individual ideas organized?
- If outlined, what would the theory look like?
- Do relationships expand concepts into larger wholes or vice versa? Do they link concepts in a linear fashion?
- Does the structure move concepts away from or toward the purposes?
- Are there several structures that emerge? What is their form? Do they fit together?
- Could more than one structure represent the overall structural relationships?
- Where is there no structure?

6. Assumptions
- What assumptions underlie the theory? Are assumptions explicit, implicit, or derivable from context and meanings?
- What are the individual, nurse, society, environment, and health assumed to be like?
- Do assumptions have an obvious value orientation? What is it?
- Could assumptions be factually verified?
- Where are assumptions located within the structure? Prior to, within, or following theoretic reasoning?
- Can assumptions be hierarchically arranged or otherwise ordered?
- Do assumptions have any identifiable relationship to theoretic relationships or structure?
- Are there competing assumptions?

those that are explicit. Often discerning relationships and structure is a prob-
lematic area in describing theory, but these traits will be present in the work
if it is a theory.

Forming a complete description of theory requires systematic and critical
examination of the work. Often every word, phrase, and sentence must be examined and reexamined for meaning. Ideas that emerge in response to the
descriptive questions often lead to uncertainty and revisions of earlier ideas.
After a time, the description does begin to take shape, and fewer changes occur. There will always be some tentativeness in your descriptions because your
description requires your own interpretive insights with respect to the theorist's ideas and these insights change. If you are not able to reach a tentative
resolution with respect to the fundamental nature of a theory after reasonable
study and thought, the best course of action is to propose your ideas for revision and further development of the theory. Your continuing uncertainty indicates that further theoretic development must occur.

ADDITIONAL ELEMENT OF DESCRIPTION: SCOPE

For some purposes, it may be important to describe the breadth or the scope
of the theory. Scope is not a structural component of theory per se, but it can
be considered a structural trait. It is sometimes important to describe the
scope of theory because its scope reflects its usefulness for practice and research purposes. Also, traditional typologies for describing theory such as *micro* and *macro* require knowing the scope of the theory. The purposes and
concepts are key elements when the scope of theory is described.

The scope of a theory refers to the breadth or range of phenomena to
which the theory applies. The level of abstraction of the concepts of the theory is integral to its scope. Theory may be characterized as *micro, macro, molecular, midrange, molar, atomistic,* and *holistic. Grand theory* is a term also found in
the literature, meaning theory that covers broad areas of concern within a discipline. *Meta theory* is a term used to designate theory about theory and the
processes for developing theory.

Categorizations of scope are relative, and labels that are typically used to
classify the scope of theory reflect a continuum of breadth. Micro, molecular,
and atomistic, for example, suggest relatively narrow-range phenomena,
whereas macro and molar imply that the theory covers a relatively broader
range of phenomena. These categories are often relative to the scope of the
discipline. What is micro for one discipline may be midrange in others. A theory of holistic humans would likely be broad in scope in almost any discipline
and would deal with patterns reflecting the whole. Grand theory, unlike macro
and molar theory, refers to very broad-scope theory in most disciplines. The
term *atomistic* implies a narrow scope and has the connotation of assuming that

parts are a legitimate focus for study in order to generalize about the whole. Conversely, holistic connotes that the sum of parts cannot reflect the whole.

Figure 6–3 depicts these theory classifications relative to each other on a breadth continuum. There are no predetermined criteria for determining whether a theory is micro, macro, molecular, midrange, or molar. At best, these words are guides.

Two descriptive components of theory can be used as a basis for determining where a theory is placed in terms of breadth: purpose and concepts. For theoretic purposes ask, How broad are they? The following illustrate a narrowing scope of purpose:

- Consciousness expansion
- High-level wellness
- Illness recovery
- Pain alleviation
- Regional blood flow improves
- Amplitude and frequency of action potential on nerve fiber bundles increase

Micro or molecular theory may reflect purposes that can only be known indirectly because evidence to validate their achievement requires perceptions keener than those provided by unaided senses. The purpose of altering action potential is representative of this category. Improving regional blood flow is an even broader purpose than altering action potential, since in some cases it is indirectly perceptible, whereas action potentials cannot be assessed without sensitive signal processing equipment. Concepts contained in such theories are narrow and often specifically defined.

When the purpose increases in scope to represent a portion of an accepted overall purpose for a profession or discipline, midrange theory is

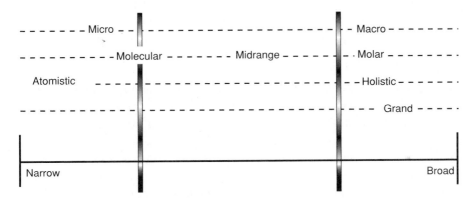

FIGURE 6–3 Relative classification of theory based on breadth of concepts and goal statements.

being approached. Theory of pain alleviation is an example of this range, because pain alleviation is one of several areas of concern to nursing. Micro theories might attempt to explain the physiology of pain phenomena, whereas midrange theories would deal with pain alleviation as a segment of nursing's total interest. Concepts contained in midrange theory reflect this part of whole orientation; they are broader than those contained in micro theories but still do not reflect the totality of nursing's concern.

Macro theories conceptualize purpose broadly. Health, expanded consciousness, and high-level wellness, not just for individuals but for people in general, are examples of such purposes. Macro theories deal with the whole of nursing's concern. Concepts within these theories tend to be broad in scope and related to individuals as wholes rather than as portions of the person's structure or function.

An example may serve to illustrate how purpose and concepts interrelate to provide information that can be used in responding to questions about scope. Abdellah and her colleagues (1960) have proposed that nursing purposes can be described as the solution of problems in twenty-one different categories. Each problem is complex in itself, and taken together they are represented as the totality of nursing function. Problem 11 is "to facilitate maintenance of sensory function." Theory regarding the solution and prevention of sensory function as a problem could be considered midrange theory, since it is only one of twenty-one others of concern to nursing. Narrower theory is possible concerning the development or maintenance of sensory function in diverse groups such as those with chronic illness, the young or aged, or any of numerous subdivisions. Theory of sensory neural transport would represent micro theory in relation to this problem area. Assume that the maintenance of function in all twenty-one problem areas constitutes health, whereas the solution of existing problems constitutes movement from illness toward health, with health being a valued purpose for individuals. Macro theory would be theory that interrelates all twenty-one problem areas so that the general purpose of health restoration or maintenance could be approached.

As awareness of the implications of theory for practice emerged, nurse scholars have increasingly turned attention to developing midrange theory as the desired scope for nursing theory. Some midrange theory is grounded in existing macro- or molar-level nursing theory. Others derive primarily from nursing practice, where a micro-level problem gives rise to more generalizable, but relevant, insight. Regardless of the breadth that is desired or sought, the purpose should help achieve an accepted nursing purpose. If the goal is to alleviate pain, theory and research that focuses on nerve action potentials can be justified with respect to its link to the nursing practice goal of alleviating pain.

Broad purposes may be achieved by linking narrower theories or by initially formulating broad theory. The assumptions and values orientation underlying both approaches differ. Many persons believe that a reductionistic approach (linking parts to explain the whole) is not desirable. Others state that molar theories are not useful for directing research or practice and must be reduced before laboratory testing and practice application. Given the range and complexity of nursing's purposes, a range of breadth or scope of theories is needed.

CONCLUSION

Theory can be described on the basis of its purpose, concepts, definitions, relationships, structure, and assumptions. Describing theory requires careful study of the work and interpretive responses to questions concerning descriptive elements of the theory. Each of these components is derived from the definition of theory used within this text. Once theory is thoughtfully described, critical questions can be addressed that reveal ideas concerning its function. These questions are considered in Chapter 7.

REFERENCES

Abdellah FG et al: Patient-centered approaches to nursing, New York, 1960, The Macmillan Co.
Hall LE: Another view of nursing care and quality. In Straub KM and Parker KS, editors: Continuity of patient care: the role of nursing, Washington DC, 1966, Catholic University Press, pp 47–60.

7

Critical reflection of nursing theory

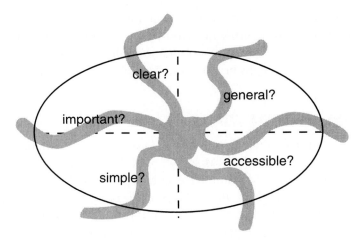

Critical reflection is a process that asks how
well a theory serves a purpose. The nature of
theory, as revealed with critical reflection, is basic to
choosing theory to guide research, practice, and education.

Describing and critically reflecting theory are fundamentally different processes. Description can be compared to setting forth facts about the theory or asking, What is this? Critical reflection, on the other hand, involves ascertaining how well a theory serves some purpose. Critical reflection is a process that asks, How does it (theory) function or work? For what purpose?

In this chapter, we identify questions that can be used in critical reflection. As you question how a theory works, you will form insight that will help you know how theory might be used and how it might be further developed.

QUESTIONS FOR REFLECTION

As you study and read different nursing theories, you may have thoughts like, "This does not seem right," or "Maybe I could do this," or "This is really exciting." When these types of thoughts occur, what you are doing is comparing the theory to some personal and perhaps unrecognized ideas about what is important for theory. Each nurse's ideas of the adequacy of a theory are influenced by a personal perspective of what is valuable or good. For *research*, you might agree: "This could be helpful." For *practice*, you might think: "Maybe I could use this." For *idea stimulation*, you might think: "This is really exciting." In these instances, you have formed an impression of the value of the theory from personal values about practice, research, and critical thinking. Your own values are important components that contribute to a more formal critical reflection process.

Critical reflection contributes to understanding how well the theory relates to practice, research, or educational activities. Members of a discipline form ideas about what questions to ask and what responses are generally accepted if a theory is to be seen as valuable for the discipline. Just as there are many ways to describe theory, there are many critical questions that can be asked about the functional value of theory and many responses to these questions. Once the questions are asked, members of a discipline can consider what responses they tend to value and why. The questions we suggest are organized around characteristics of theory. These characteristics form the basis for considering the merits and shortcomings of a theory in relation to some purpose. The questions we pose are consistent with generally accepted methods for evaluating theories that have been described in the nursing literature (Ellis, 1968; Fawcett, 1993; Hardy, 1974; Stevens-Barnun, 1994). A theory is examined with respect to each of the questions, and the responses to the questions are used to form conclusions about how well the theory serves some purpose.

The questions for critical reflection are

- How clear is this theory?
- How simple is this theory?
- How general is this theory?
- How accessible is this theory?
- How important is this theory?

There are no correct answers to these questions, and the questions do not imply the responses. For example, the question, How clear is this? does not necessarily mean that a theory should be perfectly clear. Rather, the people who address the question use it as a tool to focus on issues of clarity and gain understanding of how this might contribute to the theory's function for a particular purpose. As you engage in discussions that are centered around the questions, you can form a consensus with your colleagues as to where to go next in developing the theory. These insights can best be formed in discussion among people with diverse perspectives. For example, even though a theory that challenges assumptions about practice is somewhat unclear, it may be an important theory for changing nursing practice and for providing new concepts with which to work. The fact that it is not perfectly clear leaves room for imagining new possibilities, which may be part of its strength.

Although each of the five critical reflection questions is fundamentally different, you will find that they are interrelated. For example, one question addresses accessibility, and another addresses generality. If a theory is seen as general or broad in scope, it may be less accessible (less related to empiric reality) than if it were narrower in scope (less general).

Responses to the description questions in Chapter 6 affect your responses to the critical reflection questions. For example, to decide how clear, accessible, or general a theory is, you need to describe some purpose of the theory, what concepts are included, and how they are structured. As your description of theory is formed, you can begin the process of critical reflection. The ideas you develop from this process contribute to your own critical insights, and to substantive discussion that gives direction for further theory development.

How clear is this theory?

In addressing this question, you will be considering semantic clarity, semantic consistency, structural clarity, and structural consistency. Clarity, in general, refers to how well the theory can be understood and how consistently the ideas are conceptualized. Semantic clarity and consistency primarily refer to the understandability of theoretic meaning as it relates to concepts. Structural clarity and consistency reflect the understandability of connections between concepts within the theory and the whole of the theory.

Semantic clarity.   The definitions of concepts in the theory are an important aspect of semantic clarity. Definitions help to establish empiric meaning for concepts within the theory. If concepts are not defined or are incompletely defined, the empiric indicators for the idea become less clear. When concepts are clearly defined, identification of empiric indicators is relatively easy. Clarity implies, in part, that when different nurses read the theory, a similar empiric reality comes to mind when the word for the concept is used. If there are no definitions or if only a few of the concepts are defined, clarity will be limited.

Types of definitions that are used within theory affect semantic clarity. When definitions reflect both specific and general traits, clarity is enhanced, whereas a general or a specific definition alone often limits clarity. Specific definitions lend clarity because they provide clear and accurate guidance for the intended empiric indicators for a concept. General definitions contribute a contextual sense of meaning for concepts, lending a richness of meaning that is not possible when concepts are specifically defined. Considering the extent to which each type of definition contributes to clarity of meaning can help you form your own ideas about the adequacy of the theory for your purpose.

Clarity may be obscured by borrowing terms from other disciplines or by using common language terms that carry broad general meanings. Words such as stress or coping have general common language meanings, and they also have specific theoretic meanings in other disciplines. If words with multiple meanings are used in theory and not defined, a person's everyday meaning of the term is often assumed, rather than what is meant in the theory; therefore, clarity is lost. Clarity is enhanced when the concept is defined consistently with common meanings of the term within the profession.

Clarity is affected when words are used that have no common meaning or when words are invented or coined by the theorist to represent some idea. Coined words can help to convey a meaning for which there is no word, but they can also detract from clarity, especially when a more familiar word or phrase would suffice. It would be possible to generate an entire theory about quizzendroids, plankerods, and ziots. The theory could be logical and consistent but unclear because the words are invented and have no meaning. Although this is an exaggerated example, it demonstrates the effects on clarity when vague or strange words are used, when words are not defined, or when words with many possible meanings are used and not defined.

Semantic clarity can also be affected by excessive verbiage. Normally, varying words to represent similar meanings is a writing skill that can be used to avoid overuse of a single term. But, in theory, if several similar concepts are used interchangeably when one would suffice, there is excess verbiage, and the clarity of the presentation of the theory is reduced rather than improved.

In theory, varying the word for important concepts interjects subtly different meanings. For example, interchanging the words *restoration, rehabilitation,* and *recovery* for the same concept changes clarity, since each word has a slightly different meaning and suggests different contexts of use.

Clarity is also affected when excessive narrative is included. Semantic clarity may be decreased by use of excessive examples; however, the judicious use of examples usually aids clarity. Diagrams can enhance or obscure clarity. To enhance clarity, diagrams should be self-explanatory and simple in expression, because overly complex illustrations discourage comprehension. In general, the alternate mode of providing information in the form of diagrams will help make the ideas in the theory clearer.

Economy of words, key definitions, and wise use of examples and diagrams lend clarity. Absolute semantic clarity can never be achieved, nor is it necessarily desirable. Because of the limitations of language, no matter how clearly the theorist represents theoretic meaning, it will not be perceived uniformly by all readers.

Semantic consistency.   Semantic consistency is a second feature to consider with respect to the question of clarity. A theory that is inconsistently presented leads to confusion. Semantic consistency means that the concepts of the theory are used in ways that are consistent with their definition. Sometimes a definition is explicitly stated, and somewhere within the theory another meaning is implied. When key words are not explicitly defined, their implied meanings may be inconsistent from one usage to the next. Occasionally, words are explicitly defined but in different ways. Inconsistencies that occur when terms are defined explicitly are fairly easy to uncover, but other types of inconsistencies may be more covert.

The consistent use of basic assumptions is important in achieving consistency. The theory's purpose, definitions of concepts, and relationships need to be consistent with the stated assumptions of the theory. Examples and diagrams can also be considered in light of the assumptions of the theory. Suppose, for example, a basic theoretic assumption is the unity of persons and environment and that both change simultaneously and irreversibly through time and space. This assumption is consistent with a definition of health as expanding consciousness but inconsistent with a theoretic conceptualization of health as a state of adaptation. Adaptation typically implies conforming or adjusting to environmental stimuli in order to fit within the environment. The concept of adaptation tends to suggest the assumption that events external to the person are primary as a determinant of health and that the person and the environment are separate entities. Unity of person and environment is a concept that can be used to convey an assumption that humans and environment are interconnected and change simultaneously. Simultaneous change negates the idea of conforming or adjusting to a stimuli as health; rather, it implies incorporating change, becoming a different person, and increasing options and awareness of choice.

For clarity, the purposes of the theory must be consistent with all other components. A purpose of health, achieved by deliberate nursing actions, may be at odds with the basic assumption that health is deterministic. The purpose in this example is to create something that is assumed to be deterministic and therefore cannot be influenced by deliberate acts. Becoming aware of this inconsistency helps to clarify other meanings that are conveyed in the definitions and other components of the theory.

In reflecting on consistency, examine your descriptions for each component of theory and consider where there are consistencies and inconsistencies within, as well as between, the descriptive elements of the theory. Definitions must be examined for consistency with each other and in relation to assumptions. Structure is sometimes inconsistent with relationships. If a theory is extremely inconsistent, it is difficult to continue the process of critical reflection concerning the theory. Some semantic inconsistencies within theory are more common early in their development and leave room for new possibilities for further development. However, inconsistencies at the basic roots of theory, as between assumptions and goals, have implications that will affect the entire theory and must be addressed.

Structural clarity.   Structural clarity is closely linked to semantic clarity. Structural clarity refers to how understandable the connections and reasoning within theory are. The descriptive elements of structure and relationships provide important information for addressing this dimension of clarity.

In a theory with structural clarity, you can readily recognize the underlying conceptual network. With structural clarity, concepts are interconnected and organized into a coherent whole. If you cannot discern the structure of the theory, you begin to search for those structural elements that are related and for gaps that occur in the flow of the theory. If all major relationships are included within a single structure, clarity is enhanced. Clarity is lost if the relationships are not contained within a coherent structure. Pieces of relationships, rudiments of structure, or concepts that stand alone are evidence that parts have not yet been integrated into the whole during the development of the theory.

Structural consistency.   Structural consistency relates to the use of different structural forms within theory. Usually theory is built around one predominant structural form. Sometimes one form provides the general profile for the conception of the relationships of theory, and subcomponents of the theory

take a somewhat different form. Whatever the structure, consistency throughout the theory with respect to the structure serves as a conceptual map that
enhances clarity. A theorist may begin with a structural movement that is linear. If this structure is reflected in the relationships as the theory develops,
you will observe a high level of structural consistency. A shift in reasoning to
a structure of differentiation may be confusing, or the reasoning might function well within the overall structure.

In summary, the question, How clear is this theory? can be used to explore in what ways a theory is clear and comprehensible, how it is not, and
what its level of clarity means for the development and use of the theory. The
ideas of semantic and structural consistency and clarity can be used to guide
discussion of issues of clarity. A very general (broad scope) theory may be
quite ambiguous but useful in stimulating new ideas. A midrange theory of
hopelessness, for example, may have aspects that are vague but still be important in helping nurses understand the experience. However, the ambiguity of that same theory may affect its usefulness for guiding research.
Becoming aware of the ways in which clarity is obscured in light of your purpose makes it possible to design ways to further develop its clarity. The degree
to which a theory must be clear depends on how the nurse intends to use it.

How simple is this theory?

Complexity implies many theoretic relationships between and among numerous concepts. On the other hand, theoretic simplicity means that the
number of elements within each descriptive category, particularly concepts
and their interrelationships, are minimal.

The following example illustrates theoretic simplicity. Suppose that a theory contained three major concepts: A, B, and C. A theory interrelating these
concepts would be quite simple, since only three interrelationships would be
possible: A and B, A and C, and B and C. Adding subconcepts 1 and 2 to A,
B, and C (e.g., A1, A2) would leave the theorist with three major concepts (A,
B, and C) and six subconcepts, for a total of nine. A theorist working with
nine concepts has significantly greater theoretic complexity than a theorist
working with only three concepts. Adding even one or two concepts to a theory greatly increases potential for theoretic interrelationships and, subsequently, complexity.

The desirability of simplicity or complexity varies with the stage of theory
development. In grounded theory, for example, there may be considerable
complexity as the theory begins to emerge, but, as it develops, relationships
and concepts are coalesced, and the theory becomes more simple. Regardless
of approach to theory development, some concepts created early in the
process may eventually be deleted or changed. In the above example, suppose

concepts A, A1, and A2 came to be seen as unimportant in relation to the theory's purpose. The theoretic complexity added by A and its subconcepts could be removed, and only the simpler relationships between B and C and their subconcepts would remain.

Theories reflect varying degrees of simplicity. In nursing, some situations suggest the need for relatively simple and broad theory that can be used as a general guide for practice. Other situations suggest simple but more empirically accessible theory to guide research. Still other situations suggest the need for theory that is relatively complex because of the value such theory has for enhancing understanding of extremely complex practice situations.

How general is this theory?

The generality of a theory refers to its breadth of scope and purpose; a general theory can be applied to a broad array of situations. *Parsimony* is sometimes used as a synonym to describe the trait of theoretic simplicity, but the concept of parsimony also includes the idea of generality. A parsimonious theory is conceptually simple (contains few structural elements) but accounts for a broad range of empiric experiences.

The scope of concepts and purposes within the theory provide clues to its generality. A theory containing broad concepts will encompass more ideas with fewer words than one containing very narrow concepts. Concepts of humans and universe could be interpreted as organizing almost every fact or idea possible. A comprehensive theory with these two concepts would be highly generalizable. A theory interrelating the individual and the physical environment is less general, although still fairly broad in scope. The concept of individual implies that the theory is concerned with a single person. The use of *physical* as a modifier for *environment* conveys the notion of environment in part only. Information about individuals in communities could not be understood within this theory. A theory relating characteristics of acutely ill people with the intensive care unit environment is even less general, and the scope of concepts narrows.

Questions that address the generality of theory include To whom does this theory apply, and when does it apply? Is the purpose one that pertains to all health care professionals? To people in general? Does the purpose apply to specific specialties of nursing and only at given times? The more limited the scope of application of the theory, the less general the theory.

Whether or not generality is viewed as desirable depends on your purpose for the theory. General theory organizes many ideas and is quite useful for generating ideas or hypothesis. Nursing theories that address broad concepts, such as individuals, society, health, and environment, have a high degree of generality and are useful for organizing ideas about universal health behaviors.

Theories that address a specific human experience such as pain are less general and, because of their relative specificity, are useful for guiding practice in a clinical setting.

How accessible is this theory?

Accessibility addresses the extent to which empiric indicators can be identified for concepts within the theory and how attainable the projected outcomes of the theory are. If a theory is to be used for explaining and predicting some aspect of the practice world, its theoretic concepts must be linked to empiric indicators available in practice. Concepts can move toward increased empirical accessibility through generating and testing relationships, deliberately applying the theory, and clarifying conceptual meaning.

Only selected dimensions of highly abstract concepts may be empirically accessible. If the concepts of a theory do not reflect empiric dimensions or if the empiric dimensions are very obscure, they may be ideas that cannot be explored or understood empirically.

Consider an example of a theory about rehabilitation and interaction. The theoretic definition of the concepts are clues to the accessibility of the theory. Without definition, the words *rehabilitation* and *interaction* can assume many dimensions of meaning. If the concepts are defined, how they are to be empirically accessed is made clearer. If definitions do not clearly suggest their empiric basis, and the purpose of the theory is to promote rehabilitation, an empiric basis for rehabilitation must be located within a clinical context.

Increasing the complexity within theories often increases empiric accessibility. As subconceptual categories are clarified, empiric indicators become more precise. Suppose that the concepts of rehabilitation and interaction are related within the same theory. The theory has a high degree of generality and simplicity, since the concepts are broad and few in number. Complexity can be increased by designating five subconcepts for each. Those five subconcepts are likely to have a more precise empiric basis than the broader concepts. With empirically accessible subconcepts, the empiric accessibility of the theory increases. If a concept does not have an empiric basis at the outset, specifying subconcepts for larger wholes does not increase empiric accessibility.

Research testing both requires and establishes the empiric accessibility of concepts. For example, if rehabilitation is defined operationally in a research project as "attainment of 70% of full range of motion," you have established a clear link between the idea—rehabilitation—and a reasonable clinical observation. If the research supports the hypothesis derived from the theory, it also provides evidence of empiric accessibility for the concept of rehabilitation.

Empiric accessibility of concepts contained within theory is basic to testing theoretic relationships and deliberately applying the theory. Grounded approaches to generating theory assume empiric accessibility. The extent to which empiric accessibility is important can vary. Considering what the theory is developed to do will help you make judgments about how empirically accessible a theory should be. Theory that provides a conceptual perspective of clinical practice may not need much empiric accessibility. If a theory is to be used to guide research, empiric accessibility is important. If a theory is to be used to shape nursing practice, concepts need to be empirically accessible in the clinical area. If concepts are not empirically grounded, concept clarification may be used to provide direction for empiric indicators needed for research.

How important is this theory?

In nursing, the importance of a theory is closely tied to the idea of its clinical significance or practical value. An important theory is forward-looking, useful, and valuable for creating a desired future. The central question is Does the theory create a reality that is important to nursing? Many realities will be important to nursing. Some nursing theory guides research and practice, some generates radically new ideas about health and caring, and some differentiates the focus of nursing from other service professions.

If a theory contains concepts, definitions, purposes, and assumptions that are grounded in practice, it will have practical value for enhancing theory-based research. A theory that has limited empiric accessibility may not have practical value for research but can stimulate ideas and spark political action that improves practice.

One approach to addressing the question of importance is to reflect on the theory's basic theoretic assumptions. If underlying assumptions are unsound, the importance of the theory is minimal. If, for example, a theory is based on a view of the individual as parts, its importance for nursing is minimal. If a theory is based on an assumption of holism, and it moves understanding of holism to a new dimension, it is likely to be highly important to nursing.

Theories that have extremely broad purposes may be essentially unattainable and therefore have limited value for creating clinical outcomes. This same theory may be important for generating ideas and challenging practice.

The importance of theory will depend on professional and personal values of the person who is addressing the question. Asking the questions, Do I like this theory? and, Why? will help identify the values you hold for your self, your practice, the profession, and the theory. Contributing your ideas about what is important for nursing through careful deliberation and discussion among nurse colleagues will help discern the direction for a theory to achieve important professional purposes.

GUIDE FOR THE CRITICAL REFLECTION OF THEORY

How clear is this theory?

- Are major concepts defined?
- Are significant concepts not defined? Are definitions clear? Congruous? Consistent?
- Are words coined? Are coined words defined?
- Are words borrowed from other disciplines and used differently in this context?
- Is the amount of explanation appropriate? Too much? Not enough?
- Are examples or diagrams helpful? Not helpful? Needed and not present?
- Are examples and diagrams used meaningful?
- Are basic assumptions consistent with one another? With purposes?
- Is the view of person and environment compatible?
- Are the same terms defined differently?
- Are different terms defined similarly?
- Are concepts used in a manner consistent with their definition?
- Are diagrams and examples consistent with the text?
- Are compatible and coherent structures suggested for different parts of the theory?
- Can the theory be followed? Can an overall structure be diagrammed?
- Where, if any, are gaps in the flow? Do all concepts fit within the theory?
- Are there any ambiguities as a result of sequence of presentation?
- Does the theorist accomplish what she/he sets out to do?

How simple is this theory?

- How many relationships are contained within the theory?
- How are the relationships organized?
- How many concepts are contained in the theory?
- Are some concepts differentiated into subconcepts and others not?
- Can concepts be combined without losing theoretic meaning?
- Is the theory complex in some areas, not in others?
- Does the theory tend to describe, explain, or predict? Impart understanding? Create meaning?

How general is this theory?

- How specific are the purposes of this theory? Do they apply to all or only some practice areas? When?
- Is this theory specific to nursing? If not, who else could use it? Why?
- Is the purpose justifiably a nursing purpose?
- If subpurposes exist, do they reflect nursing actions? How broad are the concepts within the theory?

Continued.

GUIDE FOR THE CRITICAL REFLECTION OF THEORY—cont'd

How accessible is this theory?

- Are the concepts broad or narrow?
- How specific or general are definitions within the theory?
- Are the concepts' empiric indicators identifiable in reality? Are they within the realm of nursing?
- Do the definitions provided for the concepts adequately reflect their meanings?
- Is a very narrow definition offered for a broad concept? A broad meaning for a narrow concept?
- If words are coined, are they defined?

How important is this theory?

- Does the theory have potential to influence nursing actions? If so, to what end? Is that end desirable?
- Does the theory influence nursing education? Nursing research? If so, to what end? Is that end desirable?
- How specific are the purposes of the theory? Do they provide a general framework within which to act or a means to predict phenomena?
- Is the theory's position about people, about nursing, and about the environment consistent with nursing's philosophy?
- Given the purpose of the theory and its orientation, what of significance for nursing or health care has been omitted?
- Is the stated or implied purpose one that is important to nursing? Why?
- Will use of the theory help or hinder nursing in any way? If so, how?
- Will application of this theory resolve any important issues in nursing? Will it resolve any problems?
- Is the theory futuristic and forward-looking?
- Will research based on the theory answer important questions?
- Are the concepts within the domain of nursing?
- Do I like this theory? Why?

FORMING A COMPLETE CRITICAL REFLECTION

In summary, the five questions for critically reflecting a description of theory are

- *Is this clear?* This question addresses the clarity and consistency of presentation. Clarity and consistency may be both semantic and structural.
- *Is this simple?* This question addresses the number of structural components and relationships within theory. Complexity implies numerous relational components within theory. Simplicity implies fewer relational components.
- *Is this general?* This question addresses the scope of experiences covered by theory. Generality infers a wide scope of phenomena, whereas specificity narrows the range of events included in theory. Generality combined with simplicity yields parsimony.
- *Is this accessible?* This question addresses the extent to which concepts within the theory are grounded in empirically identifiable phenomena.
- *Is this important?* This question addresses the extent to which theory leads to valued nursing goals in practice, research, and education.

The list of questions presented in the box on pp. 135–136 provides a guide for forming critical reflections of theory.

CONCLUSION

The critical reflection of theory in relation to clarity, simplicity, generality, accessibility, and importance will guide the development of theory so that it is in harmony with an envisioned future. The nature of theory, as revealed with critical reflection, is basic to choosing theory for guiding research, practice, and education. In Chapter 8, we present a discussion of interrelationships between theory and research.

REFERENCES

Ellis R: Characteristics of significant theories, *Nurs Res* 17(3):217–22, 1968.
Fawcett J: Analysis and evaluation of conceptual models of nursing, ed 3, Philadelphia, 1993, FA Davis Co.
Hardy ME: Theories: components, development, evaluation, *Nurs Res* 23(2):100–107, 1974.
Stevens-Barnum BJ: Nursing theory, ed 4, Boston, 1994, Little, Brown & Co.

8

Nursing theory and research

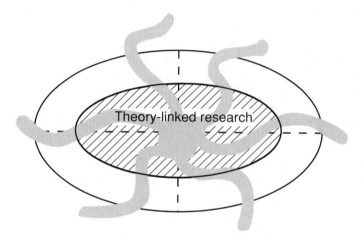

Philosophic commitments of researchers,
the philosophy of nursing, and the emerging
theory are integral to the choices the researcher
makes about method. Deliberate choices that link
research methods, theory, and practice are basic to empiric knowledge that assists nursing to achieve valued goals.

I n this chapter, we examine the relationship between theory and research.
Although standard research texts describe the basic standards that
guide the research process and the different types of research approaches
that fit within these standards, the assumptions underlying the standards are
not usually stated explicitly. Moreover, the philosophic commitments of the
researcher, the fundamental philosophy of the discipline, and the theory that
is emerging consistent with that philosophy are integral to the method and to
choices the researcher makes about method. In this chapter, we introduce
ways in which research choices can be designed or evaluated to be theoretically sound.

THEORY-LINKED RESEARCH AND ISOLATED RESEARCH

Research is the systematic application of the methods of empirics in order to
develop knowledge. Research can be used as a means to test theoretic relationships and as a method to generate concepts or relationships for the construction of theory.

Of all of the processes of theory development, research-related activities
are more visible to the casual observer than the cognitive-based theoretic
processes. The concept of research is often associated with an image of a laboratory where experiments are conducted or where some activity occurs that
involves discovering facts. Actually, creating empiric knowledge is more related to theory than it is to uncovering isolated facts that can be reported in
great detail and numbers. Factual knowledge is useful, but facts alone are insufficient for developing empiric knowledge. In order to develop empiric
knowledge, facts must be interpreted in relation to one another and conceived as having meaning (Bleich, 1978; Greer, 1969; Scheffler, 1967; Silva
and Rothbart, 1984).

Research, like theorizing, can be conducted in a variety of ways and with
multiple motivating factors. There are many descriptions of different types of
research, and each research text presents a somewhat different way of viewing
the total process. The traits of each approach that are common reflect certain
basic standards that have been established in order to obtain results that are
considered reliable and valid or accurately representative of empiric reality.
Two types of research can be conducted in accord with accepted standards—
theory-linked or *isolated research*. The major trait that distinguishes theory-linked
research from isolated research is that theory-linked research is designed to

develop or test theory. It is this quality that sets the stage for the study to contribute to the larger knowledge of the discipline. Isolated research, on the other hand, is not linked to the processes of theory development.

From a research point of view, theory-linked and isolated research can both be of excellent quality. Both types of research can ultimately contribute to knowledge, although isolated research is much more limited in the contribution it can make to a discipline. Because theory-linked research is conceived and conducted within the framework of theory, the findings of research have greater potential for contributing to the development of useful knowledge.

In isolated research, the investigator formulates questions or hypotheses and uses accepted methods to refute or support the hypotheses or to answer the questions. Questions or hypotheses may come from the practical circumstances surrounding the investigator's work, the imagination, an idea that occurred in reading other research results, or any number of other sources. These same factors can also provide direction for the development of theory-linked research.

Research is confined to a particular place and a time in history. Since theories are constructions of the mind, they can transcend, to a certain extent, these limitations. The cultural and historical circumstances of the theorist influence the mental construction of the theory, but because the theory is an abstraction, it is possible to move beyond the limits of particular circumstances. Isolated research, which often focuses on particulars of a specific problem, offers little potential for speculating about the significance of the research beyond what can be justified by the method, design, and analysis of study results. The results of isolated research can provide new insights that prompt the researcher, or someone reading the report of the research, to speculate about larger implications of the research for the discipline, which in turn can lead to developing theory that has broader meaning for the discipline.

Theory-linked research has advantages that overcome the limitations of the specific place and time in which the research occurs. Theory-linked research hypotheses that are developed from abstract statements of the theory represent a translation of the theory's abstract statements to the circumstances of the specific study. These research findings can only be generalized within limits, just as those reported in isolated research. However, the study findings in theory-linked research can be retranslated to theoretic terms and implications discussed in relation to the theory.

Problems of theory-linked research

Although theory-linked research has definite advantages over isolated research in being able to contribute to the development of knowledge, certain hazards and problems are unique to this type of research.

Inappropriate use of theories.   It is possible to use a theory inappropriately in conducting research. For example, if a theory is designed to explain animal behavior, it may not be appropriate as a basis for explaining human behavior, and vice versa, without sufficient conceptual examination. Theory and theoretic concepts that are used inappropriately lead to erroneous conclusions. Reed (1978), for example, describes how some theories in behavioral sciences have resulted in erroneous information concerning primate behavior. Using theories of human behavior, primate sexual behavior has been categorized as either monogamous or polygamous. On the basis of limited observations of animal behavior, it became common practice to describe animal behavior using these terms. Reed (1978, p. 49) points out that, in reality, animals seldom cohabitate on the basis of sex differences, and segregation of male and female primates is more pronounced than cohabitation. Theories sometimes provide a mental set that clouds observations, especially if the theory is assumed to be true or consistent with prevailing values.

Theories as barriers.   Theories can obscure the ability to notice certain features or events. This is because the set provided by theory, whether appropriate or not, may preclude recognition of other possibilities. When the focus is on expected outcomes, unless something startling or drastically different occurs, some elements may not be noticed. For example, you can view a child's behavior and, because of a certain theory, assume that what you observe is problem-solving ability. At the same time, you might fail to notice other things about the child's behavior because they are not brought to your attention by the theory. These other behaviors might include less obvious and therefore easily overlooked actions such as body posture, facial expressions, or eye motion. It is possible that qualities of these behaviors relate to problem-solving ability, but the mental set that you acquire from the theory focuses your attention on limited behaviors, and something potentially important in understanding the child's reality is overlooked.

Paradoxically, although a theory may be useful and appropriate for understanding reality, it may limit your thinking about the range of possibilities and experiences. Overcoming this difficulty requires that you constantly question what you read, think, and observe. Theory is not intended to represent exact truth or reality; it is intended to be an approximation and a tool to see new possibilities. The purpose for using research to develop theory is to discover to what extent a theory can be regarded as sound and to what extent it functions to open new possibilities.

Ethical considerations.   Theories can also exceed acceptable limits of reality; theories as mental constructions may relate ideas that cannot or should not be tested, out of respect for human and animal rights and dignity. For example, given the threat of nuclear accidents, you might imagine that it would be useful to predict events in a large population of people who experience a significant exposure to radiation. This knowledge might help in preparing for this circumstance. In reality, it is not ethical to subject humans or animals to such an experience to develop theory. Nor is it feasible to test an armchair theory developed to predict the consequences of exposure to radiation.

Occasionally, historical circumstances provide evidence that is used to develop useful theory, but further testing is limited by concern for human and animal welfare. Theories of mother-infant attachment and separation grew out of the experiences of wartime children separated from their mothers for extended periods of time. The evidence that grew out of the historical disaster was amply sufficient to demonstrate the harmful effects, and further research that replicates similar circumstances is ethically indefensible.

THE RELATIONSHIP BETWEEN THEORY AND RESEARCH

In this chapter, our focus is on theory-linked research processes and on examining how empiric research contributes to theory development. One way of viewing this relationship between theory-linked research and theory is as a spiral (Fig. 8–1). The spiral represents the interaction between theory and research. If you begin with theory, research derived from the theory is used to clarify and extend the theory. If you begin with research, theory that is formed from the findings can be subsequently used to direct research. In order for this spiral process to continue, research must be conducted with the specific aim of contributing to theory development.

The processes of generating and testing theory, as well as deliberately applying the theory, draw on research methods. Research also provides information that can be used in creating conceptual meaning and in structuring and contextualizing theory. There are essentially two ways in which research is linked to theory development: by generating theory and by testing theory.

(1)   (2)

Theory-generating research

Research that generates theory is designed to discover and describe relationships without imposing preconceived notions of what these phenomena mean. This is usually thought of as an inductive approach. It is impossible to observe events in the real world without some preconceived mental image of what they mean. Preexisting mental images are inherent in the experience of being socialized in a human culture; the process of learning the theories of a discipline conveys meanings. When a researcher designs a study to generate theory, observations are made with as open a mind as possible in order to see things in a new way.

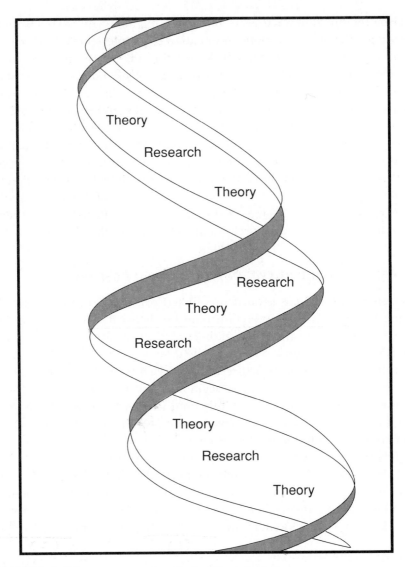

FIGURE 8–1 Theory-research spiral of knowledge.

As an example, suppose that a marketing analyst wanted to develop a theory about what motivates people to buy certain items. If the analyst decided to use a theory-generating approach, her research could begin by observing the shopping behavior of people in a mall. The analyst would probably already have some belief that advertising does affect behavior based on theories of behavior and marketing. Her perceptions during the observation would not be really pure but would be influenced by theoretic notions about how people shop. However, if the intent of the theory builder is to try to discover some previously unaccounted for variable or to describe something about shopping behavior that has not been described, preconceived ideas about this behavior must be recognized and set aside as far as possible.

One approach to theory-generating research that has been used in nursing is grounded theory (Glaser and Strauss, 1967). This is a form of field methodology that requires the simultaneous processes of collecting, coding, and categorizing empiric observations and forming concepts and relationships based on the data obtained. Grounded-theory methodologies also use deductive approaches to examine propositions of theory. However, it is initially an inductive method.

Other forms of theory-generating research include field observations, as used in anthropology, and participant observation, as used in sociology. The investigator attempts to minimize any intrusion or effect on events observed and seeks to view and describe things occurring as they would if the observer were not present. The investigator attends to clues about how one event affects another and explains the things observed by developing theoretic relationship statements about those observations (Stern, 1980).

Since many phenomena cannot be observed directly, theory-generating research must sometimes use indirect ways of gathering data. Phenomenology is one example of this approach. Phenomenology as a research method is designed to describe the subjective, lived experiences of people and to comprehend the meanings that people place on these experiences (Omery, 1983). These are experiences that cannot be observed; they are directly accessible only to the person who has the experience. Indirect ways of observing empiric reality include interviewing or questioning individuals about what they feel or remember or how they respond to certain situations. Feelings, thoughts, memories, dreams, and private human experiences can only be observed through how people choose to relate them.

Different inductive methodologies produce different types of knowledge and different forms of descriptive statements or theories. Grounded-theory methods result in relationship statements or propositions that the researcher has observed in empiric experiences. Phenomenology results in interpretive narratives that describe meaning as fully as possible. Regardless of the approach, inductive investigators whose purpose is to contribute empiric knowledge for the discipline systematically organize and describe their research results, often in the form of a proposed theory.

Theory-testing research

Once theory is constructed, by whatever means, it is possible to use research methods for validation. The methods are designed to ascertain how accurately the theory depicts phenomena and their relationships. Theoretic statements can be translated into questions and hypotheses as long as the abstractions of the theory can be represented with empiric indicators. A single study is usually based on one or two relational statements from among several that might possibly be extracted from a theory. No one study can test the entirety of a theory. Some theories contain some relationship statements that can be tested and other relationship statements that cannot be tested using research because empiric indicators cannot be identified.

Even though a theory has been incompletely tested, it is generally regarded as relatively sound if several research studies conducted over time in different settings demonstrate a degree of confidence in the theory. If some statements are supported by research, whereas others are unsupported or refuted by research, the research provides a basis for revising the theory or developing new theory.

Theory-testing research is usually thought of as a deductive approach. The research starts with an abstract relational statement derived from theory. From the theoretic statement, hypotheses or research questions are created for a specific research situation.

Research questions may also be used in theory-testing research. This type of research typically uses descriptive and correlational designs. The concepts in the research questions are empirically represented, and observations are made. The data are collated and described in such a way that the questions are addressed, and implications related to the development of the theory are stated.

Since hypotheses must contain a relationship between at least two variables, the research design is usually an experimental, quasi-experimental, or correlational approach (Polit and Hungler, 1987; Shelley, 1984). In theory-testing research, the investigator deliberately changes or controls conditions so that the study clearly focuses on the nature of the relationship between the variables that have been selected for study. Several descriptive and relationship testing studies are needed to eventually test a theory, since only a limited number from among all possible relationships can be included in one study. A single study can contribute appreciably to the validation process if it is theoretically sound.

In the following sections, we examine the general research process and identify how both theory-generating and theory-testing research can be designed and therefore evaluated to achieve the most value from the research effort.

DEVELOPING SOUND THEORETIC RESEARCH

The research process can be examined for theoretic soundness at each stage. The following descriptions of each stage can serve as a guide for developing or evaluating the theoretic soundness of a research study. Examples are given in each section from two research studies to illustrate features of theory-testing and theory-generating research. The example of theory-generating research used an emergent design, grounded-theory approach, and ethnographic interviewing strategies to generate a hypothesis concerning parents' perceptions of the meaning of quality nursing care for hospitalized children (Price, 1993). The example of theory-testing research used a repeated measures analysis of variance technique to analyze perceived pain thresholds of women with chronic pain during and after listening to music of their choice (Schorr, 1993).

The clinical problem, research purpose, research problem, and hypotheses

In theory-linked research, the purpose, the problem statements, and the hypotheses are designed to show the relationships between the chosen theory base and the particular study being conducted. In theory-testing research, each of these statements should be explicitly formulated, because they direct movement from the broad, general intent to the empiric specifics of the study. In descriptive and exploratory theory-testing research, hypotheses may not be stated or labeled as such, and research problems (questions) are developed. Although not necessarily stated in relationship form, the questions imply underlying relationships of significance to the developing theory.

In theory-generating research, only the clinical and the research problems are required; the other statements may or may not be developed explicitly in the course of the research process. These are not necessarily explicitly stated in published reports of completed research, but in well-reported studies, the statements appropriate to each approach can be inferred from the text of the published article.

In theory-testing research, statements of purpose, problem, and hypotheses or questions are formulated in advance of conducting the data-gathering activity. In theory-generating research, the purpose and problem statements are formulated in advance; if relationships are stated, they are derived from the data. Table 8–1 describes the purpose served by each type of statement and shows how clinical problem, research purpose, research problem, and hypotheses follow from each other and provide a conceptual link between the theory and the research study.

As the table shows, there are two types of problems: clinical and research. The clinical problem is a question that reflects the general experiential concern that generated or influenced the study and suggests the study context. The clinical problem does not specify or imply relationships but simply indicates the context within which theoretic relationships will be generated or tested.

TABLE 8-1 Comparison of clinical problem, research purpose, research problem, and hypothesis statements in theory-linked research

Type of statement	What the statement conveys	Theory-generating*	Theory-testing*
Clinical Problem	Specifies the experiential observations that generated or influenced the study.	How do parents of hospitalized children perceive their care?	What can be done to alleviate chronic pain?
Research purpose	Specifies whether the research is theory-generating or theory-testing.	To generate substantive theory that explains parental perceptions when their children are hospitalized.	To test music as a unitary-transformative means of altering the perception of chronic pain within the context of Newman's theory (1986) of health as expanding consciousness (Schorr, 1993, p. 31).
Research problem	Poses a question to be answered. Is less general than the purpose and makes clear how the purpose is to be achieved. Expresses the nature of the variable or events to be studied. Implies the empiric possibilities for the abstract concepts given in the purpose.	What does quality nursing care mean to parents of hospitalized children (Price, 1993, p. 35).	Does music change the pain perception threshold?

TABLE 8–1 Continued

Type of statement	What the statement conveys	Theory-generating	Theory-testing*
	Expresses the relationships between concepts if the relationship is the focus for the study.		
Hypothesis	Indicates the specific choices made in relation to the variables for the study. Implies the design of the study. Implies the type of analysis used.	Quality nursing care involves a process of parent and child interaction with the nurse that leads to the establishment of a positive relationship and ultimately results in the satisfaction of the biopsychosocial needs of the parent and child (Price, 1993, p. 40).	The pain perception threshold will increase with the use of music as a unitary-transformative nursing intervention (Schorr, 1993, p.31).

*Sources: Pauline J. Price, "Parents' Perceptions of the Meaning of Quality Nursing Care," *Adv Nurs Sci* 16(1):33–41, and Julie Anderson Schorr, "Music and Pattern Change in Chronic Pain," *Adv Nurs Sci* 15(4):27–36, 1993.

The research purpose indicates whether the study is theory-generating or theory-testing in nature and whether the study focuses on description, explanation, or prediction. If the study is for the purpose of generating theory, the purpose further states the empiric reality the investigator is studying. If the study is theory testing, the purpose states the theoretic frame of reference for the study.

For both theory-generating and theory-testing research, the research problem is less general than the statement of purpose and directs the more specific, circumstantial focus of the study. The research problem is phrased in the form of a question that implies how the purpose of the study is to be achieved. It reflects the variables or events to be studied and implies that empiric possibilities for abstract concepts to be developed are embodied in existing theoretic relationships.

When hypotheses are stated, they indicate the circumstantial restrictions of the study, reflect the study design, and suggest the analysis to be made of data. Hypotheses usually provide specific guidance for statistical analysis of quantitative data. If the analysis of the research data does not depend on statistics for drawing conclusions, hypotheses might not be stated; rather, research questions are used to guide data analysis.

In theory-generating research, hypotheses may or may not be stated. Problem statements or research questions may be appropriate for guiding a study intended to generate theory, and hypotheses are formulated at the conclusion of the study, if at all. When formulated, hypotheses provide specific direction for future research.

Background of the study and literature review

In all research, the literature review surveys research findings that are pertinent to the study being conducted. In theory-linked research, the literature review also includes a summary evaluation of the theoretic background for the study.

For theory-generating research, the background for the study includes a review of previous writings, including the theoretic, philosophic, and empiric studies pertinent to the area of concern. The author's thinking and experience are important as background for the study. The literature review is not necessarily completed in advance. As the ideas and concepts emerge from the data, the researcher uses the data to guide explorations in the existing literature. The empiric observations remain the primary source for analysis and interpretation, but in some instances the literature provides a basis for refining and delineating central concepts and the relationships between them.

In theory-testing research, previous studies based on the theory form a substantial portion of the literature review. The review also contains a critique of previous research based on alternative theories and on concepts or variables shown to be related to the study's central purpose. The review traces how the study has been conceived and summarizes the theoretic ideas that are being tested. This clarifies how and why specific relationships within the theory are being tested.

In Table 8–1, Schorr's study (1993) is used to show how statements of clinical problem, research purpose, research problem, and hypotheses are formulated. In this study report, the background includes a description of Margaret Newman's (1986) theory of health as expanding consciousness that formed the basis for study. The background focuses on explaining the way in which the study variable (music) was conceptualized as patterned environmental resonance that may precipitate a shift in consciousness. The variable of pain pattern of rheumatoid arthritis was viewed as an evolving pattern of the whole, with action potentials to be uncovered. The related literature provided evidence that substantiated the notion that music as patterned environmental resonance influences the interconnectedness of the entire living system.

Price's report (1993, p. 35) drawing on grounded theory as an emergent design (one approach to theory-generating research) illustrates the conception of a research idea from questioning how consumers view quality of care. The literature they reviewed substantiated that nurses and consumers tend to view quality differently but that there is little evidence on which to base understanding of consumer perspectives of quality. The author was convinced that nurses need to understand the client's perspective of quality in order to be recognized as providers of quality, cost-effective care. From Price's perspective, the existing literature on consumer perspectives of quality of care offered insufficient background for building and influencing the development of concepts and theoretic relationships that could inform the development of quality nursing care. She also notes that most of the literature that addresses consumer satisfaction with care relies on quantitative studies based on instruments designed and compiled by health care providers, which inserts the bias of the provider in the results that are reported.

The research method

Several concerns with regard to research method must be carefully considered when theory-linked research is undertaken. These include the means of obtaining the data, the selection of the sample for study, the design of the research, and the analysis of data and conclusions.

The means of obtaining data.   How the data are collected or recorded must be consistent with the purpose of the research design. For theory-generating research, the study is usually descriptive in nature and requires either directly or indirectly observing and recording empiric events that the investigator does not alter during the course of study. Theory-testing research also draws on these means of obtaining data. Because this type of research often relies on some type of experimental or correlation analysis, the tools used tend to be those that yield quantitative measures of the variables.

Direct observation requires being physically present. Data are recorded by some means, such as note taking, audio taping, or videotaping. Examples include watching and making notations about behavior during the processes of mother-infant interactions, about interactions between nurses and clients within an intensive care unit, or about behavior of a person experiencing a crisis such as pain.

Indirect observation includes the following: interviews; questionnaires and standardized tools that elicit feelings, thoughts, or memories; or self-reports of experiences not directly observable. Tools designed to elicit reports about selected phenomena must be carefully examined to be sure they can provide the evidence needed to achieve the purposes of the study. Tools developed with a particular theoretic bias introduce a perspective that may not be desirable in theory-generating research. Paradoxically, a tool developed to explore several possibilities regarding the reality of an experience may be needed for theory-generating research yet may lack the reliability and validity needed for accurate results. In theory-testing research, the means of obtaining data must be carefully considered in relation to theoretic adequacy of tools and measurement approaches. In both types of research, the problems of reliability and validity of both direct and indirect observations are considered. Tools that are designed to yield a numeric score are assessed for reliability and validity using statistical methods. Tools and interview approaches that are designed to produce narrative descriptions are examined carefully to ascertain how well the approach will function to elicit the type of responses that are needed. The research report should include a discussion of the level of development for the tools used, what theoretic perspective underlies any tools used, and what evidence exists of the tool's reliability and validity.

In Schorr's study (1993), the McGill Pain Questionnaire was used to measure women's perceived pain thresholds. The author discusses the pain-rating indices that provide a pain-rating intensity measure and a pain-rating index. Schorr cites literature evidence that supports the tool as a reliable and valid indicator of clinical pain. In addition, she discusses issues concerning the measurement of fatigue and energy levels and the approaches that other researchers have taken. She concludes that it is reasonable to measure energy levels by asking people to express differences in their experiences of energy.

In Price's study (1993) of parents' perceptions of quality nursing care, ethnographic interviews and field notes were the methods used to obtain data. The interviews were audiotaped and transcribed.

The selection of the sample.   The selection of the sample is essentially what limits the research to a particular time and place. It is a part of the research that links the abstractions of the theory with empiric phenomena. In theory-generating research, the investigator begins with the following assumption: "There is some phenomenon or event happening in reality that will be evident if I observe this particular group of people. Furthermore, this particular group is sufficiently like other groups of people who have this experience to represent them." The individuals chosen for the sample are purposely selected because they can contribute information and insight related to the phenomenon being studied.

In theory-testing research, sample selection requires the investigator to take the position that if the theory being tested is empirically reasonable, it will be supported by what happens with the specific persons selected for study. Or, if the theory is not empirically accurate, the responses of the sample studied will refute the theory. Since most theory-testing research relies on statistical analysis of quantitative data, sample selection is guided by the requirements of statistical analysis. Both the population to whom the theoretic relationship applies and the sample that is being tested must be specified. Drawing the conclusion of empiric accuracy of the relationship depends on the assumption that the statistical requirements for sampling from the identified population have been met.

In Price's study (1993) of parents' perceptions of quality of care, the four parents of hospitalized children composed a convenience sample. Since the study was exploratory in nature, no other restrictions were placed on the sample selection process.

In the report of Schorr's theory-testing study (1993), the sample consisted of thirty women who were diagnosed with rheumatoid arthritis for a minimum of six months were solicited from the practices of private physicians. They were all able to read and speak English and were capable of giving informed consent. The criterion for sample selection was consistent with Newman's theory (1986) on which the study was based; that is, both health and disease are manifestations of the evolving pattern of increasing complexity.

The research design.   The design of the research outlines the procedure and contingencies used for answering the research questions or testing the hypotheses. In theory-generating research, the design must be consistent with the theory-generating orientation of the research. This often involves observation of a particular kind of phenomenon of interest in given groups. Stern (1980) describes the design of grounded theory as a matrix in which several research processes are in operation at once. The investigator examines obtained data and begins to code, categorize, conceptualize, and write impressions about its meaning.

Sometimes, research designs that are typically used in theory-testing research are needed for theory-generating research. This is the case when a sequence of ordinarily occurring events is an area of concern. For example, suppose something happens to create a sequence of events, such as the birth of a child or the death of a loved one. The research interest might be to describe the usual responses of individuals over a period of time, both before and after this event, in order to generate theory regarding how people live through these situations. In these instances, comparative assessments over time are needed. The investigator does not, as in classic experimental designs, impose the changes as a part of the design but rather waits for the changes to occur. The investigator then describes the nature of outcomes occurring before and after the event in order to develop theory.

Theory-generating research also may require comparison groups that are typical of experimental designs in order to determine if a phenomenon occurs only under certain circumstances. Suppose, for example, that an investigator wanted to determine if body image formation were appreciably affected by chronic illness. The phenomenon could be studied by comparing body image formation in a group of people having a chronic illness with body image formation in a group not having chronic illness. The comparison would determine if aspects of the phenomenon of body image formation were unique to people with chronic illness. This information would contribute to the development of theory related to body image formation.

In some forms of theory-testing research, the researcher deliberately alters circumstances in some way to test the relationships expressed in the hypotheses. The design usually includes some intervention or investigator-created circumstances consistent with the theoretic basis for the study.

In Schorr's theory-testing study (1993), a repeated-measures design was used to test the effects of music on perceptions of pain. The researcher or the participant provided a cassette tape of the woman's favorite type of music. Participants completed the McGill Pain Questionnaire and then listened to the music for an uninterrupted period of twenty minutes. At the end of the period of music, participants again completed the questionnaire, and at the end of another two hours, completed the questionnaire again.

In Price's study (1993) of parents' perceptions of quality of care, the grounded-theory approach was selected for two reasons—because methods to study perceived quality of care that rely on instruments constructed by health care providers carry the bias of the provider, and because there was a need to accurately conceptualize phenomena that occur within the nursing domain. The grounded-theory approach provides a continuous and interactive process that promotes a fit between what people actually experience and the theory that emerges as a result of coding that experience. This approach also provides for conceptualizing a phenomenon that is clearly within nursing's domain but that had not been adequately described in the literature.

Analysis of the data and conclusions.   The analysis of data in theory-linked research must be consistent with the purposes of the research and the research design. For theory-generating research, analysis of data involves narrative, descriptive, and other relatively qualitative types of analysis. Depending on the type of observation used, a quantitative, numeric, or statistical analysis of the data can also be presented, but this is accompanied by a theoretic analysis that includes the full range of observations and the ways in which the observations occurred.

In a grounded-theory approach, analysis of the data involves coding and categorizing the observations. In participant observation, the analysis may report sample observations that typify the characteristic events or the sequence of events that was observed. Whatever the form of data presentation, the investigator proposes concepts generated from the data and, if possible, a description of theoretic propositions that emerge from the data. The extent to which concepts and theoretic propositions are formulated depends on how well the evidence supports making conceptual and theoretic formulations and on the extent to which previous studies support such conceptual and theoretic development.

In theory-testing research, analysis of the data should present sufficient quantitative and qualitative evidence to support or reject the hypotheses or to address the research questions. The conclusions of the study should include an interpretive analysis of the findings in relation to the theory being tested. The analysis of data focuses on the specific study findings, whereas the conclusions focus on the theoretic significance of the study.

In Price's grounded-theory method (1993), the data analysis involved coding transcriptions from taped interviews and field notes and examining the units of analysis for patterns through the technique of constant comparative analysis. Patterns were then analyzed for new categories and concepts. The relationships among the categories and concepts gave form to the emergent hypothesis of the study. The process of data analysis led to the following summary of the substantive process:

> Preliminary theory development suggests that what parents experience as quality nursing care involves a four-stage process: maneuvering, the process of knowing, forming positive relationships, and receiving quality nursing care (Price, 1993, p.37).

In Schorr's theory-testing study (1993), numeric data from the responses to the McGill Pain Questionnaire were analyzed using repeated measures analysis of variance for each dimension measured on the questionnaire. Results indicated statistically significant differences in perceived levels of pain before listening to the music and after listening to the music. Specifically, the pain perception threshold increased for a period of time after listening to the music. Schorr (1993, p. 34) interprets this finding theoretically in terms of patterned environmental resonance that may enable women to move beyond their pain at least for the duration of the music. The findings of the study support the research hypothesis of the study.

Generalizability and usefulness of the study

In theory-linked research, one of the important considerations for a single study is how it contributes to theory development. In most instances, a single study raises more questions than it answers, and questions raised must be presented in order to provide a basis for future study. Theory-generating research should result in relationship statements that can be studied and used in further developing the theory. Theory-testing research may result in evidence that suggests revision or extension of the theory tested, or it may suggest an entirely new avenue for development of theory.

Theory-generating research is often immediately useful for practice because of its grounding in the experience for which the theory is designed. Theory-generating research often also provides a basis for further theory-related work based on new insights and new questions. Theory-testing research can also have immediate practice application. If the research design is valid and the findings are generalizable and consistent with related research findings, the investigator may conclude that certain approaches in the realm of practice might be useful. However, immediate use in practice cannot always be expected. The primary value of theory-testing research is to stimulate further study and theory development that will add to empiric knowledge on which practice can be based.

CONCLUSION

Theory-linked research may be either theory-generating or theory-testing. Research approaches can be used to test theoretic relationships and formal application of theory and can contribute to the structuring of theoretic relationships. Links between research and theory are basic to empiric knowledge that assists in achieving valued nursing goals. In Chapter 9, we consider the relationships between theory and practice.

REFERENCES

Bleich D: Subjective criticism, Baltimore, 1978, Johns Hopkins University Press.
Campbell DT and Stanley JC: Experimental and quasi-experimental designs for research, Chicago, 1963, Rand McNally & Co.
Glaser B and Strauss A: The discovery of grounded theory, Chicago, 1967, Aldine Publishing Co.

Greer S: The logic of social inquiry, Chicago, 1969, Aldine Publishing Co.

Newman, MA: Health as expanding consciousness, St. Louis, 1986, Mosby-Year Book, Inc.

Omery A: Phenomenology: a method for nursing research, *Adv Nurs Sci* 5(2):63, 1983.

Polit B and Hungler B: Nursing research, ed 3, Philadelphia, 1987, JB Lippincott Co.

Price PJ: Parent's perceptions of the meaning of quality nursing care, *Adv Nurs Sci* 16(1):33–41, 1993.

Reed E: Sexism and science, New York, 1978, Pathfinder Press.

Scheffler I: Science and subjectivity, Indianapolis, 1967, The Bobbs-Merrill Company, Inc.

Schorr JA: Music and pattern change in chronic pain, *Adv Nurs Sci* 15(4):27–36, 1993.

Shelley SI: Research methods in nursing and health, Boston, 1984, Little, Brown & Co.

Silva MC and Rothbart D: An analysis of changing trends in philosophies of science on nursing theory development and testing, *Adv Nurs Sci* 6(2):1–13, 1984.

Stern PN: Grounded theory methodology: its uses and processes, *Image* 12(1):20–23, 1980.

9

Nursing theory and practice

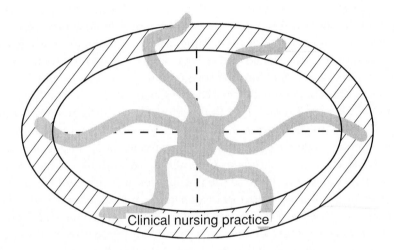

Clinical nursing practice

If theory is expected to benefit practice, it must be developed cooperatively with people who practice nursing. People who do research and develop theories think differently about theory when they consider the reality of practice.

There are important relationships between nursing practice and the processes of theory development. Theories do not provide the same type of procedural guidelines for practice as do situation-specific principles and procedures or rules (Beckstrand, 1980). Procedural rules or principles help to standardize nursing practice and can be useful in achieving minimum goals of quality of care. Theories exist to challenge existing practice, create new approaches to practice, and remodel the structure of rules and principles.

One way that theory challenges existing practice is that it provides new ways to think about problems, which makes it possible for practitioners to envision new approaches to practice. Since theories are not sets of rules, but are tentative, practice also challenges theory. The processes of theory development as described in Chapter 5 depend on the continual tests of the practice perspective. Nurses who do research and develop theories learn to think differently about theoretic problems and issues as they perceive the realities of practice. Nurses who practice on a day-to-day basis also learn to think differently about their practice as they contribute to the possibilities of theory and research.

By *nursing practice*, we mean the experiences a practicing nurse encounters during the process of caring for people. Some experiences are those of the client, others are those of the nurse, some are interactive, and some are environmental. These experiences may also occur in other settings, but, when they occur in the context of providing nursing care, they are considered part of nursing practice.

In this chapter, we address specific ways in which practitioners can contribute to theory development processes. One avenue is through the process of creating conceptual meaning, which brings together the practical and the theoretic to benefit both practitioner and theorist. The deliberative application of theory also provides specific opportunities for practicing nurses to make critical decisions regarding when and how to apply theory in practice and how to judge the effect of the theory's application on the broader goals of nursing practice. Although nurses use theory in practice in many different ways, in this chapter we consider how practice contributes to and benefits from processes of creating conceptual meaning and deliberately applying the theories.

CREATING CONCEPTUAL MEANING

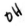

Concepts do not simply appear or arise; they develop from perceived experience. The perceptual experiences from which nursing concepts develop are found in the practice of nursing. Practicing nurses who reflect on the nature of their experiences make significant contributions to theory development. Individuals who are primarily involved in theory development benefit from the ideas of many nurses who practice nursing. Individuals do not participate equally in all processes required for the development of theory; rather, individual nurses participate in a collective endeavor.

➤ Empiric concepts are formed from nursing practice by observing, naming, and making sense of what happens. A concept is not the experience itself. The mental image that develops from the experience and the language that is used to convey the idea make it possible for practitioners and others to communicate about that experience. Concepts are generally ambiguous, particularly to an experienced practitioner who prefers precise guides for practice. But, even with ambiguity, concepts provide a mental tool for quickly comprehending a range of specific experiences and thinking about what those experiences mean. Once concepts are integrated into theory, the theory provides explanations that bring to awareness interpretations of specific situations.

The processes of creating conceptual meaning (described in Chapter 5) can be used as ways to draw on experiences in nursing practice that contribute to theory development. One approach is to present practice situations as model, related, or borderline cases for concepts. The practice situation is also useful for identifying appropriate empiric indicators for nursing concepts. The following sections describe four practice-dependent activities that contribute to the process of theory development in nursing.

➤ Identification of empiric indicators

Practice provides essential evidence that is used to select empiric indicators for abstract concepts. The experiences of practice can challenge existing theoretic conceptualizations, and they can reveal hunches that have not yet been linked to a particular concept or theory. The basic question is, What have I experienced that can be linked to the abstract concept X? Anxiety is a good example of such an experience.

Suppose that a wide range of behaviors observed in practice are described in a theory as manifestations of the concept of anxiety. These behaviors might include wringing of hands, silence and refusing to talk, excessive talking, laughing, crying, sweating, compulsive eating, or not eating (lack of appetite). Tools have been constructed that assess the concept using these empiric indicators. In your practice experience, you observe that these ideas do not always fit. When you work with individuals who are anxious, you observe that they tend to behave in ways that are not consistent with the theoretic concept. There are some behaviors that you almost never observe and others that are commonly experienced but not taken into account by the theory. Since anxiety as an abstract idea does convey something that you know exists, it might be helpful if you could better identify it, understand how it works, and determine how people experience it differently. As you draw on your experience, new ideas begin to emerge from the empiric behaviors you have noticed. This information is invaluable for the practice-sensitive theorist.

Differentiation of similar concepts

Concepts that are similar yet different might share certain empiric indicators, and differentiating them from one another may be difficult. If knowing the difference between them is important in practice, practice can provide the empiric information and conceptual insights required to distinguish one from another. This purpose becomes critical when you realize that errors can be made in assigning meaning to a person's experience. For example, you might have been taught that certain behaviors are manifestations of anxiety, based on a popular theory of anxiety. You have developed an approach to assist people who are anxious to reduce their anxiety and improve their function, but it does not seem to be as effective as you think it should be. One problem might be that the behaviors are not indicative of anxiety but are associated with another feeling. Your challenge is to begin to conceptualize anxiety more clearly, conceptualize what else might be happening, and begin to find ways to differentiate between the two or more experiences. As you question and challenge the conceptualization and the conclusions that you draw from it, you will form a basis for restructuring the concepts and form new or revised concepts that better represent nursing experience.

Identification of new concepts

Creating conceptual meaning is a process that can lead to the identification of new concepts. Model, borderline, related, and contrary cases that come from practice reflect the richness and complexity of practice. As you reflect deliberately on these situations, your insights can lead to new ideas that contribute to forming new concepts.

For example, suppose you begin to notice that there is something about how people learn in the postoperative period that does not seem to be described in any of the literature you have read. Most learning theories have been developed and tested within classroom or laboratory settings where learners are students or other types of healthy subjects. In nursing situations, the learner is often experiencing an altered health state, and the patterns of behavior that are the focus of learning in this context have not been addressed in developing concepts and theories of learning. As you reflect on your experience, you see meanings that are different from the meaning of learning in the existing learning theories. As you discuss your ideas with other nurses, you find that they have made similar observations. From this awareness, you can build a new conceptualization that, once named, can be incorporated into theory and used in practice.

Identification of criteria for nursing diagnoses

Although criteria for nursing diagnoses are not the same as criteria for a concept as used in theory development, nursing diagnostic criteria can be derived partially from criteria for a concept. Nursing diagnostic criteria take into account generally accepted standards for practice, as well as knowledge and application of many areas of theory that are pertinent to the diagnosis. Consider, for example, the nursing diagnosis, "altered parenting related to economic problems as evidenced by impaired parental-infant attachment." In practice, the purpose is to accurately identify when this occurs in order to provide effective nursing care. The phrase "altered parenting related to economic problems" implies knowledge of how economic problems affect parenting as well as knowledge of the concept of parenting—a concept less well developed in the empiric realm than theories of attachment. The phrase "impaired parental-infant attachment" implies knowledge of human attachment theory and also suggests the focus for nursing actions. When criteria for nursing diagnoses are derived in part from a concept not yet well developed, the process of creating conceptual meaning can be used to form tentative diagnostic criteria that can be tested for empiric accuracy or validity.

The criteria for the nursing diagnosis of "altered parenting related to economic problems as evidence by impaired parental-infant attachment" could include conceptual criteria for parenting. The diagnostic criteria also include value qualifiers, such as the term *altered*, that convey the value that the practitioner assigns to a situation in the process of making clinical decisions. When the parent being considered is the mother, the diagnostic criteria might be

- Visual contact between mother and infant is minimal or absent.
- Physical touching of the infant by the mother is limited to necessary touch.
- There is minimal or no vocalization by the mother directed to the infant.
- The mother's verbal expressions focus on herself (that is, concerns for her own body or image or relationships with peers, rather than expressions focusing on the infant).
- Care of the infant resembles doll play and is easily or passively given over to another caretaker.

These diagnostic criteria do not include all conceptual criteria for mothering that are given as an example in Chapter 5, but they do reflect how one set of criteria for practice relates to another set of criteria for theory development. The choice of diagnostic criteria focuses on those that can be empirically observed and measured in practice. The diagnostic criteria may or may not be sufficient to use in formal testing of the theoretic concept. Evidence of the diagnostic criteria recorded in practice does provide a basis for decisions about how research should proceed. If the purpose of creating conceptual meaning is to form criteria useful for nursing diagnosis, then traits that are observed in practice and that can be verified and assessed need to be emphasized.

DELIBERATELY APPLYING THEORY

Deliberately applying of theory involves using research methods to demonstrate how a theory affects nursing practice and places theory within the context of practice to ensure that it serves the goals of the profession. Deliberative application provides evidence of the theory's usefulness in ensuring quality of care.

Deliberately applying theory is the essence of the theory-practice relationship. Theory that addresses goals of practice provides a way to systematically develop substantial empiric knowledge within the discipline. Theory is not a quick and easy answer to a problem but rather provides knowledge and understanding to ultimately enhance the practice of nursing.

A first step is to ascertain if the theory can be applied in practice. Some theories that hold promise may not be sufficiently developed to justify their application. Others might be poorly suited to a particular practice area. The guidelines we suggest in the following section can be used to make this decision. Once you decide to apply the theory in practice, you can then design research methods to demonstrate how well the theory contributes to your practice goals through the deliberative application of theory.

HOW TO DETERMINE IF A THEORY
SHOULD BE APPLIED IN PRACTICE

We have stated that theory ought to ultimately improve nursing practice. Usually, this goal is achieved by using theory or portions of theory to guide practice. Because theory can be applied prematurely or inappropriately, it is important to consider how sound judgments regarding the application of theory in practice are made.

One of the most common ways theory has been organized for practice is in the nursing process of analyzing assessment data. Sometimes this is termed the "scientific rationale for designing nursing care plans." In practice, judgments are often made without conscious effort or explicit explanation of the basis for the judgment. If called on to do so, most nurses could cite some valid reasons for their judgments. Although the theories cited may provide an explanation that seems rational and well founded, it is important to consider how adequate the theories are as a basis for making judgments. The adequacy of theories is equally critical when they are considered as a basis for directing nursing actions.

Theory is not the only means by which nursing practice can improve, nor does theory provide the only possible basis for practice. Certain common practices in nursing have emerged from sound principles or standards based in fundamental truths that have not yet come under sufficient challenge to be a focus for theory development. As Beckstrand (1980, p. 73) has noted, "Principles of practice are shorthand ways of referring to fundamental truths to be considered and general customs to be followed." Standards of practice reflect valued actions that are generally accepted in a given situation. Principles and standards are judged by their consistent outcomes; for example, do they consistently yield desired results in practice? They are changed not by systematically challenging the standards or the principles themselves but rather by discovering another approach that better achieves the desired outcome (Beckstrand, 1980).

Theory, in contrast, cannot be assumed to predict a desired outcome and does not exist to give specific guidelines for what should be done in a given situation. Rather, theory predicts a possible relationship that can be questioned. The goal of the theory and the goals of practice should be consistent with one another, but this cannot be assumed to be the case. If the relationships predicted by the theory are inadequate or do not accurately represent reality, the theory may not be effective in achieving practice goals. Theory can be effectively used to describe, explain, and predict a phenomenon that occurs in practice but may not adequately contribute to the goals of practice if it is applied. Since any application of theory will affect practice, deliberative use of theory cannot be undertaken lightly. The questions we suggest in the following section can be used to reach an informed decision about application of the theory so that its practice value can be assessed.

Are the theory goals and practice goals congruous with one another?

To answer this question, examine the goal of the theory and compare it with the outcomes or goals that you see as valuable for nursing practice. The existing standards of practice can be used as one basis for clarifying the values on which your practice is based and the overall goals that your practice should be reflecting. Another basis for identifying practice goals is your own view of nursing and that of nurses with whom you work. If a theoretic goal would lead to a situation that is not congruous with your idea of optimal health, for example, the theory may not be one that you would want to use. Sometimes this judgment is not easily accomplished and requires a deliberate philosophic stance with regard to nursing, health, the individual, the environment, and society. For example, application of a theory may be undertaken to determine if the theoretic goal is consistent with the goal of optimal health. If the theoretic goal is adaptation and you are uncertain if this concept is consistent with your idea of optimal health, you could undertake a trial application, observe the outcomes, and then assess the consistency of the outcomes in light of your practice goals.

Is the intended context of the theory congruous with the situation in which the theory will be applied?

This question addresses how well-suited the theory is for your situation, given the general ideas of context that are stated or implied theoretically. A theory of pain alleviation, for example, may explain the processes involved in alleviating pain in any instance in which it occurs. As you become familiar with the theory, you realize that it was developed with reference to mature adults, and you work with children. You and your colleagues would need to explore how well the ideas of the theory might transfer to your own situation before you make a decision to proceed with application of the theory.

Is there, or might there be, similarity between theory variables and practice variables?

This question compares the important variables in the construction of the theory with the variables recognized to be directly influencing the practice situation. In some instances, important practice variables may not be included in the theoretic relationship statements. For example, a learning theory may not consider the health status of the learner, and the learner is assumed to be a healthy individual. If practice variables are not accounted for in the theory or if there are substantial differences between the theoretic variables and the practice variables, the theory should be applied with caution, if at all. If the theory appears to have value and satisfies the considerations of most people who will be involved in the deliberative application process, it might be applied with systematic observation of the effect on outcomes, considering the differing variables that occur in practice. Given your observations, you may have a basis to propose revision of the theory to include important practice variables.

Are the explanations of the theory sufficient to be used as a basis for nursing action?

Responses to this question must be based on expert judgment about the particular nursing actions that are implied within the theory. As an expert nurse, you may find it difficult to describe the basis on which you would judge a theory to be sufficient or not sufficient. One specific approach in forming your ideas is to examine the correspondence between theoretic and practice variables. If variables in the nursing situation are similar to those that are suggested in the theory, you can then consider the nature of the relationships between the concepts of the theory. Examine the extent to which the explanation makes sense, in light of your practice. You may feel guarded about the sense of the theory for practice, but you can see that the perspective of the theory is reasonable. In this case, the theory is probably sufficient as a basis for nursing action, but your tentativeness about it leads you to be cautious as you proceed to use it and to plan careful documentation of the relationships you observe in practice.

An example of a sufficient theoretic explanation for application in practice is the mother-infant attachment theory. Hospitalization of children has created a classic separation response in those children who are separated from their significant parent. The theory describes behaviors (variables) that are clearly observed in hospitalized children. The theory also provides explanations for this phenomenon and predictions about the effects of severe or prolonged separation. Moreover, predictions are made concerning healthy outcomes that could be expected if child and parent separation were made less intense or prolonged. The theory provides direction for the nursing actions that are needed. These are not exact actions or specific rules or principles, but the theory does suggest types of actions that reduce separation and promote attachment.

Is there research evidence supporting the theory?

One very influential source of information for deciding whether or not a theory can be applied in practice is research evidence. Sometimes, a theorist, in presenting the theory, provides research evidence to support the initial theoretic formulation. If the evidence is convincing and attracts sufficient attention in the discipline, the professional literature will report research that either validates the initial theoretic relationships or does not support the theory. Research reports often suggest limits on the range of applicability of the theory or flaws in the initial theoretic construction based on the research evidence generated.

Since theories are not unequivocally supported by research evidence, it is the responsibility of the practitioners to determine if the evidence is sufficient to justify application of the theory in practice. This judgment is best made on the basis of several research studies. If there is little or no research evidence to justify application in practice, but most of the other concerns have been satisfied, you can feel reasonably comfortable about applying the theory. In this case, you should give particular attention to observing and recording relevant information regarding corresponding theoretic and situational variables and the limits and outcomes of the theory's application in practice.

How will this new approach influence the practical function of the nursing unit?

Before applying a theory in practice, you need to consider the ways in which this approach will affect the functioning of the nursing unit and assess the potential for observing and recording factors that are relevant to the theory's application. Successful application will depend on planning for the changes that are required, including the changes that will be needed to gather the research data for deliberative application. Questions to be addressed in planning for application include:

- Do nursing personnel need to be oriented to the theory and its application?
- Does the approach require adjustments in the function or processes of the nursing unit?
- Does the approach require additional time or an adjustment in the allocation of time?
- Will the approach require new equipment or other material resources?
- What practical arrangements and materials are needed to enhance the ease and accuracy of making and recording observations?
- How will trial application affect other activities in the setting?
- Are special provisions needed for gathering and storing information?
- How will clients be informed regarding the approaches that will be used?
- How will the data that are obtained be assessed and analyzed?
- If the theoretic goal is attained or not attained, how will the results be explained or accounted for?
- Have alternative explanations been projected in order to have sufficient information to make a judgment about outcomes?
- How will the results of the experience be compiled in order to communicate them to others?

If each of these questions can be answered in such a way that application seems feasible and desirable, application is probably indicated.

QUALITY-RELATED OUTCOMES

Methods that are used in the deliberative application of theory are drawn from the methods of evaluation research (Schroeder and Maibusch, 1984; Smeltzer, Hinshaw, and Feltman, 1987). These methods depend on knowing what outcomes you wish to achieve and on having a well-planned approach for achieving the goal. In deliberately applying theory, the approach is the application of a selected theory in a particular practice situation, as described in the previous section. The evaluation research methods depend on having some means for determining what circumstances exist prior to the application and comparing this with the results following the application. Usually, factors associated with the outcomes are identified and measured before beginning and again after the approach has been in place for a specified period of time. The following sections describe quality-related outcomes that you might consider in planning deliberative application.

Professional standards of care

The standards of nursing practice that are accepted by the nursing practice unit can be the measure for assessing outcomes related to deliberately applying theory. Since standards of care often reflect minimum acceptable practice, you may consider what extensions of the standards might be desirable in assessing the effects of the theory's application on the quality of nursing practice.

Functional outcomes

Nursing goals are sometimes defined in terms of how efficiently the work of nursing is done, how cost-effective it is, or how smoothly the work of each individual coordinates with the work of others. If these factors have been identified as a problem for a particular unit, the factors that are indicative of the problem need to be clearly specified and assessed prior to applying theory. Once the baseline data are obtained and the approach based on the theory has been in place for a period of time, the measures of functional effectiveness are obtained and compared.

Nurse satisfaction

Satisfaction with respect to nursing job responsibilities can be closely related to functional outcomes. Nurse job satisfaction can be assessed by such factors as working conditions, relationships with colleagues, personal fulfillment, various types of perceived benefits, or perceived dissatisfactions. A premise underlying the selection of this type of outcome is that if nurses are satisfied with their work situation, the quality of care they provide will improve.

Quality of care perceived by the person who receives care

People who receive care can be interviewed to ascertain their perception of the quality of care. There are several aspects of perceived quality of care that can be measured, including satisfaction with specific dimensions of care, perceived benefits from the care, and perceived dissatisfactions.

Expected outcomes related to quality of life

This type of outcome concerns general and specific dimensions that the profession defines as beneficial for people who receive care. These can include general health status, alleviation of signs or symptoms, acquisition of skill and knowledge, or improved abilities to function. Often, the theory that is being used will suggest a specific outcome that is related to one or more general quality of life goals. These goals can guide the selection of the deliberative application outcome that you choose.

CONCLUSION

In this chapter, we discussed how the activities of creating conceptual meaning and deliberately applying the theory interact with practice to contribute to theory development. An individual nurse or group of nurses can select several options on how they might proceed with any of these activities, depending on the needs of their setting and clients. Having other individuals in the environment who understand and support these activities and who can give information and assistance is a tremendous asset.

Prerequisites to be considered before application of a theory in practice are discussed, and they need to be considered in order to make a sound judgment regarding application of theory. If the prerequisites are considered and application is made considering the guidelines offered here, nursing practice will indeed make a valuable contribution to theory development.

REFERENCES

Beckstrand JA: A critique of several conceptions of practice theory in nursing, *Res Nurs Health* 3(2):69–79, 1980.

Schroeder PC and Maibusch RM, editors: Nursing quality assurance, Rockville, 1984, Aspen.

Smeltzer C, Hinshaw A, and Feltman B: The benefits of staff nurse involvement in monitoring the quality of patient care, *J Nurs Quality Assurance* 1(3):1–7, 1987.

Appendix A

INTERPRETIVE SUMMARY:
Broad Theories

BROAD THEORIES DEFINING THE SCOPE, PHILOSOPHY, AND GENERAL CHARACTERISTICS OF NURSING: 1952–91

The summaries provided here are not complete descriptions or critical reflections of the theorists' works. Rather, they are interpretive descriptions of the essential features of each conceptual model. They may be used as a basis for initial comparisons of theorists' works and as a basis for selecting a particular work for further description and critical reflection.

A notation of the definitive theoretic writing precedes the summary. When theorists have multiple publications, the summaries focus on most recent ideas. The conceptual models are presented in the order shown in Table 3–6 (p. 51). The original terminology of the theorists has been retained.

H. E. PEPLAU

Interpersonal relations in nursing, 1952

The art and science of nursing, 1988

The patient is an individual with a felt need, and nursing is a process that is both interpersonal and therapeutic. Nursing is the simultaneous application of art and science. The overall goal or purpose of nursing is to educate and be a maturing force so that personality development (a new view of self) occurs. This purpose is achieved when the nurse, as a medium for change, enters into a personal relationship with an individual, the patient, when a felt need presents itself. The personal relationship in nursing provides for meeting the individual patient's needs and assists the two persons (the nurse and patient) with different goals to develop or assume congruent goals. The nurse-patient relationship occurs in phases during which the nurse functions as a resource person, a counselor, and a surrogate. There are four phases: orientation, identification, exploitation, and resolution. When a person with a need seeks help, the nurse assists in orientation to the problem. During phase one, the illness event is integrated. The person learns the facets of the difficulty and the extent of need for help. During phase one, orientating to use of services, productively exploiting anxiety and tension, and learning the limits of necessary space and freedom occur. This helps to ensure that the illness event is not repressed. When orientation is completed to a given degree, the phase of identification begins. In phase two, the patient assumes a posture of interdependence, dependence, and/or independence in relation to the nurse. The nurse assists the patient during this phase, taking into consideration the services needed and the patient's history. Identification helps assure the patient that the nurse can understand the interpersonal meaning of the patient's situation. When identification is accomplished, phase three, exploitation, begins. In this phase, the patient derives full value from the relationship by using the services available on the basis of self-interest and needs. Resolution, the final phase, occurs as old needs are met. With resolution of older needs, newer and more mature needs emerge. When needs are resolved, the person is freed from dependence on others. The maturing force of nursing is realized as the personality develops through the educational, therapeutic, and interpersonal process of nursing. The phases of the relationship are serial, and the patient assumes an active role.

During the dyadic nurse-patient relationship and greater nursing relationships with communities, many roles are assumed by nurses. These include roles of stranger, teacher, resource person, surrogate, leader, and counselor. Multiple roles occur as a result of multiple client problems and needs in individual interpersonal relationships, team functions, and variant social and professional expectations. The overall goal for professional nursing is the same as the nurse-patient dyads—to implement a process that facilitates personality development by helping persons use forces and experiences to ensure maximum productivity.

F. G. ABDELLAH, I. L. BELAND, A. MARTIN, AND R. V. MATHENEY

Patient-centered approaches to nursing, 1960

The patient and/or family present with nursing problems that the nurse helps them meet through her professional function. There are twenty-one problem categories that the nurse addresses. These are (1) hygiene and physical comfort, (2) activity and rest, (3) safety, (4) body mechanics, (5) oxygenation, (6) nutrition, (7) elimination, (8) fluid and electrolytes, (9) responses to disease,

(10) regulatory mechanisms, (11) sensory function, (12) feelings and reactions, (13) emotions and illness interrelationships, (14) communication, (15) interpersonal relationships, (16) spirituality, (17) therapeutic environment, (18) awareness of self, (19) limitation acceptance, (20) resources to resolve problems, and (21) role of social problems in illness.

Nursing problems are both overt or obvious and covert. Nurses must be aware of covert problems to meet care requirements. Overt and covert problems must be identified to make a nursing diagnosis. Identification of problems precedes solution. The nursing process is the method nurses use to establish and focus on a nursing diagnosis. The overall goal is fullest possible functioning for a client.

Individualized patient care is important for nursing. Both patients and nurses should be aware of the wholeness of clients and the need for continuity of care from pre to posthospitalization. Individualized care will require changes in the organization and administration of nursing services and education.

I. J. ORLANDO

The dynamic nurse-patient relationship: function, process and principles, 1961

The discipline and teaching of nursing process: an evaluation study, 1972

The patient is an individual with a need that, if supplied, diminishes distress, increases adequacy, or enhances well-being. Needs include requirements for implementing physicians' plans, or other innate requirements. The nurse acts to meet needs and thus alleviate distress.

Patients with needs behave verbally and nonverbally in a given manner. The nurse reacts to patient behavior by ascertaining both the meaning of the distress and what would alleviate the distress. Finally, the nurse acts to alleviate the distress. Distress can be due to (1) physical limitations, either temporary or permanent, (2) adverse reactions to the setting, such as being misinterpreted or misinterpreting, and (3) inability to communicate.

Three elements—patient behavior, nurse reactions, and nurse actions—compose a nursing situation. Patient behavior and nurse reactions relate to the assessment phase of the nursing process and involve ongoing interaction with the nurse. Once the need is clearly ascertained through assessment, the nurse acts automatically or deliberatively. Automatic actions are those carried out for reasons other than resolving an immediate need, whereas deliberative actions seek to meet assessed needs. Automatic actions make problems by creating situational conflict that is evidenced through lack of resolution of needs and cooperation (i.e., distress is not alleviated).

Deliberative action yields solutions to problems and also prevents problems. Once the nursing action occurs, the nurse evaluates patient behavior to determine if the need has been met and resultant distress has been alleviated. The overall goal is to meet needs and, through that, to alleviate distress.

E. WIEDENBACH

Clinical nursing: a helping art, 1964

The patient is an individual under treatment or care who experiences needs. Needs are requirements for maintenance or stability in a situation that may be perceived by the individual as a requirement for help, and may be met by the person or others. Also, persons may have needs and not seek help or may help themselves without recognizing a need. Needs for help are defined as measures or actions required and desired, which potentially restore or extend ability to cope with situational demands" (p. 6). Nursing is concerned with the needs that patients have for help. What the nurse does and how she or he does it compose clinical nursing. Clinical nursing has four components: (1) philosophy, (2) purpose, (3) practice, and (4) art.

Philosophy is a personal stance of the nurse that embodies attitudes toward reality, and purpose is the overall goal. The purpose of clinical nursing is "to facilitate efforts of individuals to overcome obstacles which interfere with abilities to respond capably to demands made by the condition, environment, situation or time" (p.15). This purpose is the embodiment of meeting needs for help, which implies goal-directed, deliberate, patient-centered practice actions that require (1) knowledge (factual, speculative, and practical), (2) judgment, and (3) skills (procedural and communication). Practice includes four components: (1) identification of the perceived need for help, (2) ministration of help needed, (3) validation that help given was the help needed, and (4) coordination of help and resources for help—(i.e., reporting, consulting, and conferring). The art of clinical nursing requires using individualized interpretations of behavior in meeting needs for help.

The helping process is triggered by patient behavior that is perceived and interpreted by the nurse. In interpreting behavior, the nurse compares the perception to an expectation or hope. Nursing actions may be rational, reactionary, and deliberative. A rational response by the nurse is one based on the immediate perception without going beyond to explore hidden meaning. A reactionary response is one taken in reaction to strong feelings. Deliberative actions, the desirable mode, are those that intelligibly fulfill nursing's purpose. Identification of needs for help involves (1) observing inconsistencies, acquiring information about how patients mean the cue given, or determining the basis for an observed inconsistency, (2) determining the cause of the discomfort or need for help, and (3) determining whether the need for help can be met by the patient or whether assistance is required. Once needs for help are identified, ministration and validation that help was given follow.

The practice of clinical nursing is bounded by professional, local, legal, and personal constraints. Clinical nursing practice is supported by nursing administration, nursing education, nursing organizations, and nursing research. The clinical goal is to meet needs for help, integrating the practice and process of nursing. Greater professional goals include conservation of life and promotion of health.

L. E. HALL

Another view of nursing care and quality, 1966

The patient is a unity composed of three overlapping parts: a person (the core aspect), a pathology and treatment (the cure aspect), and a body (the care aspect). The nurse is a bodily care giver. Provision of bodily care allows the nurse to comfort and learn the patient's pathology, treatment aspect, and person. Understanding, resulting from the integration of all three areas, allows the nurse to be an effective teacher and nurturer. The patient learns and is nurtured in the person (that is, in the core aspect). Nurturance leads to effective rehabilitation, greater levels of self-actualization, and self-love.

Nursing occurs during one of two phases of medical care. Phase one medical care is the diagnostic and treatment phase, and phase two is the evaluative, follow-up phase. The professional nurse's role is in phase two, and professional nursing practice requires a setting in which patients are free to learn. In phase two, the nurse's goal is to help the patient learn. Motivation to learn is assured by advocating the patient's learning goals and not the doctor's curative goals. Once patient learning goals are codetermined with the nurse and motivation therefore assured, the patient will learn, and nurturance, rehabilitation, and self-love follow. The overall goal for the client is rehabilitation, which inspires a greater measure of self-actualization and self-love.

V. HENDERSON

The nature of nursing, 1966

The patient is an individual who requires help toward independence. The nurse assists the individual, whether ill or not, to perform activities that will contribute to health, recovery, or peaceful death that the individual would perform unaided if he had necessary strength, will, or knowledge. The process of nursing strives to do this as rapidly as possible, and the goal is independence. The nurse manages this process independently of physicians. Help toward independence is given autonomously by the nurse in relation to (1) breathing, (2) eating and drinking, (3) elimination, (4) movement and posture, (5) sleep and rest, (6) clothing, (7) maintenance of body temperature, (8) cleaning and grooming of the body and integument protection, (9) avoidance of environmental dangers and injury of others, (10) communication, (11) worship, (12) work, (13) play and participation in recreation, and (14) learning and discovery. Nursing can be evaluated as a profession based on the extent to which it achieves each of these functions autonomously.

The role and functions of professional nursing vary with the situation. If the total health care team comprises a pie graph in health care situations, there are some situations in which no role exists for certain health care workers. Although there is always a role for family and patients, the pie wedges for team members vary in size according to (1) the problem of the patient, (2) the patient's self-help ability, and (3) help resources. Central to nursing that seeks to help patients toward independence is empathetic understanding and unlimited knowledge. Empathetic understanding grounded in genuine interest will lead to helping the family understand what a patient needs. The ultimate goal for the nurse is to practice autonomously in helping patients who lack knowledge, physical strength, or strength of will in growth toward independence. Because of this function, nurses will seek and promote research, education, and work settings that facilitate this goal.

J. TRAVELBEE

Interpersonal aspects of nursing, 1966, 1971

Nursing is an interpersonal process aimed at assisting individuals, families, or communities to prevent or cope with the process of illness and suffering, and, if necessary, to find meaning in the experience. Nursing's purpose is achieved through human-to-human relationships, which are established by a disciplined intellectual approach to problems combined with therapeutic use of self. Human-to-human relationships require transcending roles of nurse and patient in order to establish relatedness/rapport and respond to the humanness of others. Nursing activities are a means to establishing relatedness/ rapport and achieving nursing's purpose. Nurses' values and beliefs determine the quality of nursing care provided and thus the extent to which nurses are able to help the ill find meaning in their situation.

Illness and suffering are spiritual, emotional, and physical experiences. The nurse assists the ill patient to experience hope as a means of coping with illness and suffering. Communication, a central concept for Travelbee, implies guiding, planning, and purposely directing interaction to fulfill nursing's purpose. Communication is instrumental in establishing relatedness/rapport (knowing persons), ascertaining and meeting nursing needs, and in fulfilling nursing's purpose. Communication also implies that exchanged messages are understood. Communication techniques should enable the nurse to explore and understand the meaning of the person's communication. Establishment of the human-to-human relationship is phasic. The phases are (1) the original encounter, (2) emerging identities, (3) empathy, and (4) sympathy (1971, p. 119). In such a relationship, the needs of the person are met. Achievement of a human-to-human relationship requires openness to experiences and freedom to use personal and experiential background to appreciate and understand the experiences of others.

Health and illness may be defined subjectively and objectively. Objective criteria are dependent on cultural and societal norms, whereas subjective criteria are peculiar to the human being. The meaning of the symptoms of illness (or criteria for health) for the person is more significant than affixing a label of health or illness to its results.

M. E. LEVINE

The four conservation principles of nursing, 1967

Introduction to clinical nursing, 1973

The conservation principles: twenty years later, 1989

A person is a holistic being whose open and fluid boundaries coexist with the environment, which may be perceptual, operational, and conceptual, and is a unity who is to remain conserved and integral. He sends messages that reflect his current adaptive state. Adaptation is a method of change, and change is life process. When adaptation fails, conservation is threatened, and adaptation needs occur. Adaptive needs are reflected in messages sent.

Nursing occurs at the interface between the open and fluid boundaries of whole persons and environments. The nurse receives and interprets messages and intervenes supportively or therapeutically. Intervention is guided by the four principles of conservation: conservation of energy, structural integrity, personal integrity, and social integrity. Conservation, based on an assessment of man's adaptive needs, aids adaptation. When a patient's energy and structural, personal, and social integrity are conserved—that is, when the nurse acts therapeutically—adaptation can better occur, and man achieves a state of unity and integrity. When conservation cannot be effected in the face of overwhelming adaptation needs, death ensues. Supportive interventions are appropriate when adaptation is failing without hope of reversal, such as assisting a client toward peaceful death. The goal for nursing is the wholeness of the patient brought about by conservation in four areas when adaptive needs manifest.

M. E. ROGERS

An introduction to the theoretical basis of nursing, 1970

Nursing: a science of unitary man, 1980

Science of unitary human beings: a paradigm for nursing, 1983

Nursing: a science of unitary human beings, 1989

A unitary human being is an energy field coextensive with the universe. Human-environment boundaries are only conceptually imposed and are arbitrary. The unity of human beings and environment is plausible, considering the sameness of matter and energy. Humans are more and different from the sum of their parts, and generalities about the whole cannot be made from a study of the parts. The energy composing unitary human beings and environmental field is characterized by four dimensions in which a given point in time is not tenable. The four concepts—energy fields, openness, pattern and organization, and four dimensionality—are used to derive principles that postulate how human beings develop. These principles are (1) integrality (formerly complimentarity), (2) resonancy, and (3) helicy. According to the principle of integrality, the human and environmental fields interact mutually and simultaneously. Resonancy postulates the nature of wave pattern changes as continuous from lower frequency to higher frequency patterns. Helicy asserts that field changes are innovative, probabilistic, and characterized by increasing diversity of field patterns.

Nursing seeks to care for unitary human beings in accordance with its science and art. Science is emergent and based on research and logical analysis of the principles of homeodynamics. Nursing science seeks to describe, explain, and predict. Art is the imaginative and creative use of knowledge and science. Nursing's goal is maximization of health potentials of individuals, family, and groups consistent with health's ever-changing nature. This is achieved by artfully applying emerging science based on the principles of homeodynamics.

D. E. OREM

Nursing: concepts of practice, 1971, 1980, 1985, 1991

Orem's self-care deficit theory of nursing includes theory of (1) self-care deficit, (2) self-care, and (3) nursing system. Self-care deficit theory postulates that people benefit from nursing in that they have health-related limitations in providing self-care. Self-care theory postulates that self-care and care of dependents are learned behaviors that purposely regulate human structural integrity, functioning, and development. Nursing systems theory postulates that nursing systems form when nurses prescribe, design, and provide nursing that regulates the individual's self-care capabilities and meets therapeutic self-care requirements.

Assumptions basic to the general theory are

1. Humans require deliberate input to self and environment in order to be alive and to function.
2. The power to act deliberately is exercised in caring for self and others.
3. Mature humans will sometimes experience limitations in ability to care for self and others.
4. Humans discover, develop, and transmit ways to care for self and others.
5. Humans structure relationships and tasks to provide self-care.

Humans need continuous self-care maintenance and regulation and provide this by caring for self, which enables purposeful action. Self-care activities maintain life, health, and well-being. Health refers to the state of a person, which is characterized by soundness or wholeness of developed human structures and bodily and mental functioning. Well-being refers to a person's perceived condition of existence, which is characterized by experiences of contentment, pleasure, happiness, movement toward self-ideals, and continuing personalization.

Three kinds of self-care requisites are universal, developmental, and health deviation. Universal requirements relate to the meeting of common human needs. Developmental self-care requisites relate to conditions that promote developmental processes throughout the life cycle. Health deviation self-care requisites relate to self-care that prevents defects and deviations from normal structure and integrity and those that control the extension and effects of such defects.

Adults care for themselves, whereas infants, the aged, the ill, and disabled require assistance with self-care activities. When self-care action is limited because of the health state or needs of the care recipient, nursing responds and provides a legitimate service. Thus, patients are persons with health-related self-care deficits. Two variables affect these deficits: self-care agency (ability) and self-care demands.

Self-care agency is a learned ability and is deliberate action. Nurses, given their focus on care of patients with health-related limitations in self-care abilities, must accurately diagnose self-care agency. Thus, they must have information about deficits and their reasons for existing. Such information is basic to selecting helping methods.

Nursing agency regulates or develops patient's self-care agency and ability to meet therapeutic self-care demand. Nursing is a helping service that involves acting or doing for another, guiding and supporting another, providing a developmental environment, and teaching another. Nursing agency varies with educational preparation; orientation to practice situations; mastery of technologies of practice; and ability to accept, work with, and care for others.

Nursing systems may be wholly compensatory, partially compensatory, or supportive-educative. Wholly compensatory systems are required for patients unable to monitor their environment and process information. Such patients are unable to control their movement and position and are unresponsive to stimuli. Partially compensatory systems are designed for patients with limitations in movement as a result of pathology or injury or who are under medical orders to restrict movements. Supportive-educative systems are designed for patients who need to learn to perform self-care measures and need assistance to do so. Nursing systems are formed to regulate self-care capabilities and meet therapeutic self-care requirements.

I. M. KING

Toward a theory for nursing: general concepts of human behavior, 1971

A theory for nursing: systems, concepts, process, 1981

King's general systems framework and theory, 1989

The patient is a personal system within the environment who coexists with other personal systems. Individuals form groups that comprise interpersonal systems, and interpersonal systems contribute to social systems. Thus, patient and nurse are composed of personal systems as subsystems within interpersonal and social systems. The nurse must understand given aspects of all three systems. Concepts identified for each system affect total system function. There are three comprehensive concepts: perception for the personal system, organization for the social system, and interaction for the interpersonal system. Personal system concepts related to perception include self, body image, growth and development, time, space, and learning. The nurse also must have knowledge of role, communication, transaction, and stress to understand interactions central to interpersonal system function. Since interaction occurs within social systems—including family, belief, educational, and work systems—nurses require knowledge or organizational concepts of power, authority, control, status, and decision making in order to function adequately.

The focus for nursing is the human being in the system context. The goal is health. Health implies helping people in groups attain, maintain, and restore health, live with chronic illness or disability, or die with dignity.

Interactions of the individual with the environment are significant in influencing life and health. Nurse and patient meet in a health care organization— patient needing help and nurse offering help. Nurse and patient perceive one another, act and react, interact and transact. In this process, presenting conditions are recognized, goal-related decisions are made, and motivation to exert control over events to achieve goals occurs. Transactions are basic to goal attainment and include social exchange, bargaining and negotiating, and sharing a frame of reference toward mutual goal setting. Transactions require perceptual accuracy in nurse-client interactions and congruence between role performance and role expectation for nurse and client. Transactions lead to goal attainment, satisfaction, effective care, and enhanced growth and development. The goal of nursing process interaction is transaction, which leads to attainment of goals set in relation to health promotion, maintenance, and recovery from illness.

B. NEUMAN

The Betty Neuman health care systems model: a total person approach to patient problems, 1980

The Neuman systems model, 1982, 1989

The person is a unique, holistic system, yet possesses a common range of normal characteristics and responses. Persons are a dynamic composite of physiologic, psychologic, sociocultural, developmental, and spiritual variables. These variables interact with internal and external environmental stressors. The holistic system of the person is open. As an open system it interacts with, adjusts to, and is adjusted by the environment. The external environment is defined as all that interfaces with the person's system. The internal and external environments are a source of stressors that have different potentials to disturb the normal line of defense and disrupt the system. The normal line of defense is essentially the usual steady state of the individual and is composed of the normal range of responses to stressors within persons that evolve over time. The flexible line of defense cushions and protects individuals from stressors. Lines of resistance are conceptualized as internal factors that help persons defend against stressors, and they protect the core structure and stabilize and return individuals to a normal line of defense when stressors breakthrough.

The system's model is based on an individual's relationship to stress, the reaction to it, and reconstitution factors that are dynamic in nature. The nurse assesses, manages, and evaluates patient systems. Nursing's focus is the variables that affect a person's response to stressors. Assessment of individuals considers knowledge of factors influencing a patient's perceptual field, the meaning stressors have to patient as validated by patient and caregiver, and factors the caregiver believes influence the patient situation. Basically, nursing focuses on the occurrence of stressors, the organism's response to them, and the state of the organism. Primary prevention identifies and allays risk factors associated with stressors; it focuses on protecting the normal line of defense and strengthening the flexible line of defense. Secondary prevention is related to symptomatology, intervention priorities, and treatment; it helps to strengthen internal lines of defense. Death occurs if the basic core structure of the system fails to support the intervention. Tertiary prevention protects reconstitution or return to wellness following treatment.

Nursing acts to impede or to arrest an entropic state, or a state of disorder and disorganization. Health is a state of movement toward negentropy or evolution; it is a state of inertness free from disrupting needs. Health implies a homeostatic balance. This balance depends on free energy flow between the organism and the environment. In health, the system's normal line of defense is maintained, and the lines of resistance are intact; the basic structural elements of the system are preserved.

SISTER C. ROY

Introduction to nursing: an adaptation model, 1976

The Roy adaptation model, 1980

Theory construction in nursing: an adaptation model, 1981

Introduction to nursing: an adaptation model, 1984

The Roy adaptation model, 1989

The person is an adaptive system. System inputs include (1) three classes of stimuli (focal, contextual, or residual) that arise from within the person and the external environment and (2) the adaptation level. Adaptation level is fluid, is composed of all three classes of stimuli, and represents the person's standard or range of stimuli in which responses will be adaptive.

Inputs are mediated by the control process subsystems of cognator and regulator coping mechanisms. The regulator mechanism is an automatic neuroendocrine response, whereas the cognator subsystems represent perception, information processing, and judgments influenced by learning and emotions. Coping activity may or may not be adequate to maintain integrity. A system difficulty is present when coping activity is inadequate as a result of need excesses or deficits.

The system effectors are the adaptive modes. These modes (physiologic, self-concept, role function, and interdependence) are the form in which regulator and cognator subsystems manifest their activity.

The adaptive system (person's) output is a response that may be adaptive or ineffective. Adaptive responses are those that contribute to adaptation goals (i.e., responses that promote growth, survival, reproduction, and self-mastery). Adaptation is an ongoing purposive response. Adaptive responses contribute to health and the process of being and becoming integrated; ineffective responses do not.

Using nursing process, the nurse promotes adaptive responses in the adaptive modes during health and illness. Thus, energy is freed from inadequate coping to promote health and wellness. System responses in each mode are assessed (i.e., described using objective and subjective data [first-level assessment]). Behaviors can be assessed by observation, measurement, and interviews. A tentative judgment about whether the behavior is adaptive or ineffective is then made, and stimuli influencing the adaptive system are then identified (second-level assessment). A nursing diagnosis follows, goals are set, and interventions are selected. Goals are mutually agreed on, and a goal-setting hierarchy is proposed. Survival is a priority goal, followed by goals that promote growth, ensure continuation of the race or society, and promote attainment of full potential. Factors precipitating ineffective behavior are changed, and coping behavior (i.e., adaptation level) is broadened. The person's level of coping is continuously revised. Evaluation of interventions requires returning to the first steps in the nursing process (i.e., noting behaviors manifest by the adaptive system or person).

J. G. PATERSON AND L. T. ZDERAD

Humanistic nursing, 1976

The person is a unique being, extant in all nursing situations, who innately struggles "to know." Humanistic nursing is an existential experience of being and doing so that nurturance with another occurs. Fundamentally, nursing is a response to human need and can be described to build a humanistic nursing science.

Humanistic nursing requires that the participants be aware of their uniqueness, as well as their commonality with others. Authenticity is required—an in-touchness with self that comes in part with experiencing. Humanistic nursing also presupposes responsible choices. The ability of an individual to make choices based on authentic awareness and knowledge of such choices are concerns of humanistic nursing and cultivate moreness. Also, a commitment to the value of humanistic nursing must be present.

A nurse with the foregoing attitudes and qualities can offer genuine presence to another. Humanistic nursing concerns the basic nursing act: the response of one human in need to another. At this level, nursing is related to the health-illness quality of the human condition: nurturance toward more being.

M. M. LEININGER

Transcultural nursing: concepts, theories, and practices, 1978

Caring: a central focus of nursing and health care services, 1980

The phenomenon of caring: importance, research questions and theoretical considerations, 1981

Leininger's theory of nursing: cultural care diversity and universality, 1988

Caring is postulated as the central and unifying domain for nursing knowledge and practices. Diverse factors influence patterns of care and health or well-being in different cultures. Caring includes assistive, supportive, and facilitative acts for another individual or a group with evident or anticipated needs. Caring serves to ameliorate or to improve human conditions through behaviors, techniques, processes, and patterns. Professional nursing care embodies scientific and humanistic modes of helping or enabling receipt of personalized service to maintain a healthy condition for life or death.

Caring emphasizes healthful, enabling activities of individuals and groups that are based on culturally defined ascribed or sanctioned helping modes. Caring behaviors include the following: comfort, compassion, concern, coping behavior, empathy, enabling, facilitating, interest, involvement, health-consultative acts, health-instruction acts, health-maintenance acts, helping behaviors, love, nurturance, presence, protective behaviors, restorative behaviors, sharing, stimulating behaviors, stress alleviation, succorance, support, surveillance, tenderness, touching, and trust (1981, p. 13). Culture determines personal life or world views that are mediated through language. Contextual factors such as technology, religion, philosophic beliefs, social and kinship lines and patterns, values and lifeways, political and legal factors, economic factors, and educational factors all influence care patterns. Likewise, these factors affect care patterns and health of individuals and families, as well as groups. Diverse health systems mediate the expression of health. Nursing is one health system that overlaps with folk systems and professional health care systems.

Human caring is a universal phenomenon, and every nursing situation has transcultural nursing care elements. Caring is essential to human development, growth, and survival, and caring behaviors vary transculturally in priorities, expression, and needs satisfaction. Caring plays a more important role in recovery than cure but receives less reward. If effective, caring reflects professional concern, compassion, stress alleviation, nurturance, comfort, and protection. Nursing should provide care consistent with its emergent science and knowledge, with caring as a central focus. Caring and culture are inextricably linked, and nursing care should be culturally congruent and aimed at preserving, maintaining, accommodating, negotiating, repatterning, and re-structuring care patterns.

J. WATSON

Nursing: the philosophy and science of caring, 1979

Nursing: human science and human care, 1985

New dimensions of human caring theory, 1988

Watson's philosophy and theory of human caring in nursing, 1989

Assumptions underlying human care values in nursing are (1) care and love comprise the primal and universal psychic energy and (2) care and love are requisite for our survival and the nourishment of humanity. Caring for and loving self is requisite to caring for others. Curing is not the end to be sought but is a means to care. Nursing's ability to sustain its caring ideology and translate it into practice will determine its contribution to society. Nursing has traditionally held a caring stance in relation to patients with health and illness concerns, and caring is the unifying focus for practice in nursing. Caring has received little emphasis in the health care system, and caring values of nursing are critical to sustaining care ideals in practice. Preservation of human care is a significant issue; human care can be practiced only interpersonally; and nursing's social, moral, and scientific contributions lie in its commitment to human care ideals. The foregoing assumptions provide a rationale for developing nursing as a human science.

Humans are capable of transcending time and space and possess a spirit, soul, or essence that enables self-awareness, higher degrees of consciousness, and a power to transcend the usual self. Human life is a continuous (with time and space) being in the world. Caring, an intersubjective human process, is the moral ideal of nursing. Human care processes have an energy field and involve engagement of mind-body-soul with another in a lived moment. Illness, not necessarily disease, is a state of subjective turmoil in which self as "I" is separated from self as "me." Conversely, health is a harmony within mind-body-soul in which the "I" and "me" are aligned. A healthy person is open to increased diversity. The goal of nursing is to help persons increase harmony within mind-body-soul, which leads to self-knowledge, self-reverence, self-healing, and self-care.

Theoretic premises identified include the following. At nursing's highest level, the nurse makes contact with the person's emotional and subjective world as the route to inner self; mind and soul are not confined in time and space and to the physical universe; a nurse can access inner self through the mind-body-soul, provided the physical body is not perceived separate from the higher sense of self. The geist (spirit or inner self) exists in and for itself and relates to the human ability to be free—love and caring are universal givens; illness may be hidden from the "eyes" and requires the finding of meaning in inner experiences. Finally, the totality of experiences at the moment constitute a phenomenal field or the individual's frame of reference.

Persons strive to satisfy needs experienced in the perceived phenomenal field. These include being cared for, loved, and valued and experiencing positive regard, acceptance, and understanding. Persons also strive to achieve union, transcend individual life, and find harmony with life. All needs are subservient to a basic striving toward actualizing spiritual self and establishing harmony within mind-body-soul. Harmony is consistent with a sense of congruence between "I" and "me" self as perceived, and self as experienced, as well as congruence between subjective reality (phenomenal field) and external reality (world as is).

Caring occasions involve action and choice by nurse and individual. If the caring occasion is transpersonal, the limits of openness and human capacities are expanded. Transpersonal caring relationships depend on (1) moral commitments to enhance human dignity to allow persons to determine their own meaning, (2) the nurse's affirmation of the subjective significance of the person, (3) the nurse's ability to detect feelings of another's inner condition and feel a union with another, and (4) the nurse's history of living and experiencing feelings and human conditions and imagining others' feelings (that is, personal growth, maturation, and development of the nurse's self).

Nursing interventions related to human care are referred to as carative factors and include nurturing, forming, cultivating, and using (1) humanistic-altruistic system of values, (2) faith-hope, (3) sensitivity to self and others, (4) helping-trusting human care relationship, (5) expressing positive and negative feelings, (6) creative problem-solving caring process, (7) transpersonal teaching-learning, (8) supportive, protective, and/or corrective mental, physical, societal, and spiritual environment, (9) human needs assistance, and (10) existential-phenomenological spiritual forces. Carative factors are actualized in the human care process.

M. A. NEWMAN

Theory development in nursing, 1979

Newman's health theory, 1983

Health as expanding consciousness, 1986

Individuals are subsumed by a greater whole and are part of multiple system levels in space. Explicit assumptions are made in relation to health, pathology, and patterns. Health can encompass pathology and disease; therefore, disease and health are not continuous variables or opposites. Pathology manifests according to a preexisting unitary pattern. Thus, disease gives clues to the pattern of a person's life, and pattern is reflected in energy exchange within humans and between humans and environment. Personal patterns manifesting as disease are part of larger patterns, which are not altered when the disease is eliminated. Disease as a pattern manifestation may be considered health. The existence of disease may evoke tension, an important evolutionary ingredient. Disease is not advocated as a desirable state, but the significance of attending to the meaning of the disease is highlighted. Health is an expansion of consciousness, and pattern-manifesting disease expands consciousness.

Consciousness, the informational capacity of the system, is reflected in both the quality and quantity of responses to stimuli. Health involves developing awareness of self and environment coupled with increased ability to perceive and respond to alternatives. Movement is a central concept, a property of life. The concepts of consciousness, time, movement, and space are interrelated in that movement reflects consciousness and is an identifiable and specific individual characteristic. Time is an index of consciousness and a function of movement. Movement is the means whereby time and space become reality, and space and time have a complimentary relationship. Without movement, time and space are not real, and there is no change at any system level. Movement reflects the organization of consciousness and therefore reflects health. The implied goal is consciousness expansion and therefore health and life. Health is not a state but an experienced process.

D. E. JOHNSON

The behavioral system model for nursing, 1980

The individual patient is a behavioral system composed of subsystems. As a behavioral system, the patient's subsystems strive to maintain balance, making adjustments to factors impinging on them. Humans seek experiences that may disturb balance and require behavior modifications to reestablish balance. Behavioral systems are essential and reflect adaptations that are successful. The behavioral system is composed of behaviors that form an integrated unit. Behavioral systems maintain their own integrity, link individuals with environment, and are self-perpetuating if environmental conditions remain orderly and predictable. The multiple tasks of behavioral systems require continual system changes, including subsystem evolution. Subsystems also must be protected, nurtured, and stimulated.

Behavioral system subsystems are formed from responses or response tendencies that share a common goal and are modified by maturation and experience. Each subsystem of the overall behavioral system has a specialized task or function that can be described on the basis of that structure and function. There are four structural elements in each subsystem: (1) drive-stimulated or goal sought, (2) set or predisposition to act in a given way, (3) choices, or scope of action alternatives, and (4) behavior. Only the last structural element is observable. Seven subsystems are identified: (1) attachment or affiliative, (2) dependency, (3) ingestive, (4) eliminative, (5) sexual, (6) aggressive, and (7) achievement. The attachment subsystem responses provide security, and dependency provides for nurturance responses. The ingestive and eliminative subsystems relate to eating and excretion of waste. The sexual subsystem relates to the dual responses of procreation and sexual fulfillment. The aggressive subsystem functions to preserve the person, and the achievement system functions so that mastery of self and the environment is fostered.

Nursing problems manifest when subsystems cannot maintain a dynamic stability or when the subsystem has not achieved an optimum level of function. Anticipated problems in subsystems can be prevented, and manifest problems can be solved. The nurse acts to impose a regulatory mechanism, change structural units, and fulfil functional requirements of subsystems. The nursing act seeks to "preserve the organization and integration of the patient's behavior at an optimal level under those conditions in which the behavior constitutes a threat to physical or social health, or in which illness is found" (p. 214).

R. R. PARSE

Man-living-health: a theory of nursing, 1981, 1989

Man-living-health: a man-environment simultaneity paradigm, 1985

Nursing science: major paradigms, theories and critiques, 1987

The person is unitary—that is, an indivisible being who interrelates with the environment while cocreating health. Theoretic assumptions synthesize the concepts of energy field, openness, pattern and organization, four dimensionality, helicy, integrality, coconstitution, coexistence, and situated freedom with tenets of human subjectivity and intentionality. Assumptions (nine in the 1981 work have been reduced to three in the 1987 work) state that man is a recognizable pattern who evolves simultaneously with environment. Man-environment relationships are such that a continuity of what was and what will be unfolds in the now. Man chooses the meaning given to cocreated situations and is responsible for choices made. Unitary man is recognized by individual patterns of relating, which are cocreated in man-environment interchange. There is mutual man-environment interrelatedness as man chooses to move toward irreversible possibilities. Man experiences in multiple dimensions simultaneously and relatively. The negentropic interchange of man-environment both enables and limits becoming.

Health is an open process of becoming, an incarnation of man's choosings. As man-environment connect and separate, health is cocreated. Thus, health is a synthesis of values cocreated in open interchange with environment. Health is a continuous process of transcending with the possibles (that is, reaching beyond the actual). Health is an emergent: a negentropic unfolding. The theory of man-living-health emerges from the stated assumptions, and three principles are notable:

> (1) structuring meaning multidensionally is cocreating reality through the languaging of valuing, and imaging; (2) cocreating rhythmical patterns of relating is living the paradoxical unity of revealing-concealing and enabling-limiting while connecting-separating; (3) cotranscending with the possibles is powering unique ways or originating in the process of transforming (1987, p. 163).

Principle one asserts that reality is continually cocreated by assigning meaning to all-at-once experiences occurring multidimensionally. Imaging, valuing, and languaging serve to structure meaning multidimensionally. Principle two asserts that there is an unfolding cadence of coconstituting ways of being. Ways of being are recognized in the man-environment interchange and are lived rhythmically. Rhythms of revealing-concealing, enabling-limiting, and connecting-separating are integral in the principles. The final principle asserts that concepts of cotranscending with the possibles—powering, originating, and transforming—are man's ways of aspiring toward the "not-yet." Three theoretic structures are posited:

> (1) powering is a way of revealing and concealing imaging; (2) originating is a manifestation of enabling and limiting valuing; and (3) transforming unfolds in the languaging of connecting and separating (1981, p. 68).

P. BENNER AND J. WRUBEL

The primacy of caring, 1989

Caring is primary because it determines and constitutes what matters to people. Subsequently, caring creates possibilities for coping (p. 3), enables possibilities for connecting with, and concern for, others (p. 4) and allows for the giving and receiving of help (p. 4). Caring determines what is stressful to people and how they will cope.

Drawing on Heideggerian phenomenology, Benner posits a phenomenological view of the person central to this view of caring. The person is a self-interpreting being who is defined by the process of living and being in the world. Through the process of living, people come to possess a nonreflective view of the self and can immediately grasp the meaning of a situation. This means the people understand the meaning of a context without conscious, deliberative reflection. This immediate grasping of situational meaning—self interpretation—is possible because of the human characteristics of (1) embodied intelligence, (2) acquisition of background meaning, and (3) concern.

Embodied intelligence is the capacity of being in a situation in meaningful ways and effortlessly understanding it in relation to self. Background meanings are the cultural traditions "given" to a person from birth. These two features account for how people are in the world. Concern, the third characteristic of self-interpreting beings, accounts for why people are involved in the world in certain ways. These three characteristics are central to involvement with the world in ways that ensure people will grasp the meaning of situations in relation to the situation's meaning for them. Both nurse and client are self-interpreting beings. This view of the person as self-interpreting is central to understanding how caring and concern in nursing relate to understanding and facilitating stress-coping situations in patients.

People have both freedoms and constraints that result from the assumption that people are self-interpreting (e.g., their being is contextual or situational, and they interpret contexts in relation to self). In this view, ordinary life experiences both create and determine stress and coping patterns of people. When illness and disease inevitably occur in the course of living, life contexts change and situational meanings alter. Old self-understandings do not work, a qualitatively different form of stress occurs, and the need for new patterns of coping emerge. New coping possibilities do exist in current situations, but these are understood in the context of old habits, skills, practices, and expectations (p. 23). These new possibilities and freedoms within the present contexts and situations (like the old possibilities and freedoms that no longer work) are not readily understood by the person.

Nursing is a process of helping people cope with the stress of illness, not by following sets of prescribed rules, but by contextually dependent caring and concern. Understanding the illness experience of the patient is central to concern and caring. Illness is a central focus of nursing. Illness is not reducible to disease (cellular pathology), but it connotes human loss experiences and dysfunction precipitated by human loss. Since nursing concerns itself with the relationship between the disease process and the illness experience of self-interpreting beings, a concept of mind-body dualism is not possible.

Caring in the context of nursing depends on discernment of problems, recognizing solutions, and helping patients implement, and live, a solution. This means nursing is a moral act that goes beyond mere application of scientific knowledge. Understanding the illness experience of the person is central to helping them come to live meaningful coping processes and return to health. Being present for patients and expert interpretive skills facilitate concern as a vehicle for caring. Caring concern is central to human (nurse and patient) understanding of the situation of illness. Concern allows both the nurse and patient to be in touch with the patient's lived experience. Emotions are a particular focus for concern because they are essential to patient and nurse understanding of the context of the patient, they provide clues to what is important in the situation, and they are linked to past experiences that need to be focused on and reinterpreted in the context of the present. This reinterpretation of past experiences and of old patterns of coping with life's inevitable stresses creates new contexts, and the situated freedoms and possibilities inherent in the present are more fully illuminated. New coping options result.

Since human beings can inhabit a common world with common meanings, common stress and coping patterns will exist. Phenomenologically grounded scientific study of stress and coping would reveal those common themes, meanings, and personal concerns as a basis for understanding caring practices in nursing.

REFERENCES

Abdellah FG et al: Patient-centered approaches to nursing, New York, 1960, The Macmillan Co.

Benner P and Wrubel J: The primacy of caring, Menlo Park, 1989, Addison-Wesley.

Hall LE: Another view of nursing care and quality. In Straub KM and Parker KS, editors: Continuity in patient care: the role of nursing, Washington, DC, 1966, Catholic University Press, pp 47–60.

Henderson V: The nature of nursing, New York, 1966, The Macmillan Co.

Johnson DE: The behavioral system model for nursing. In Riehl JP and Roy Sr C, editors: Conceptual models for nursing practice, ed 2, New York, 1980, Appleton-Century-Crofts, pp 207–16.

King IM: King's general systems framework and theory. In Riehl-Sisca J, editor: Conceptual models for nursing practice, ed 3, Norwalk, 1989, Appleton & Lange, pp 149–58.

King IM: A theory of nursing: system, concepts, process, New York, 1981, John Wiley & Sons.

King IM: Toward a theory for nursing: general concepts of human behavior, New York, 1971, John Wiley & Sons.

Leininger MM: Caring: a central focus of nursing and health care services, *Nurs Health Care* 1(3):135–43, 1980.

Leininger MM: Leininger's theory of nursing; cultural care diversity and universality, *Nurs Sci Q* 1(4):152–60, 1988.

Leininger MM: The phenomenon of caring: importance, research questions and theoretical considerations. In Caring: an essential human need (Proceedings of the three national caring conferences), Thorofare, NJ, 1981, Charles B Slack, Inc, pp 3–15.

Leininger MM: Transcultural nursing: concepts, theories, and practices, New York, 1978, John Wiley & Sons.

Levine ME: The conservation principles: twenty years later. In Riehl-Sisca J, editor: Conceptual models for nursing practice, ed 3, Norwalk, 1989, Appleton & Lange, pp 325–37.

Levine ME: The four conservation principles of nursing, *Nurs Forum* 6(1):45–59, 1967.

Levine ME: Introduction to clinical nursing, ed 2, Philadelphia, 1973, FA Davis Co.

Neuman B: The Betty Neuman health care systems model: a total person approach to patient problems. In Riehl JP and Roy Sr C, editors: Conceptual models for nursing practice, ed 2, New York, 1980, Appleton-Century-Crofts, pp 119–31.

Neuman B: The Neuman systems model, Norwalk, 1982, Appleton-Century-Crofts.

Neuman B: The Neuman systems model, ed 2, Norwalk, 1989, Appleton & Lange.

Newman MA: Health as expanding consciousness, St. Louis, 1986, Mosby-Year Book, Inc.

Newman MA: Newman's health theory. In Clements IW and Roberts FB, editors: Family health: a theoretical approach to nursing care, New York, 1983, John Wiley & Sons, pp 161–75.

Newman MA: Theory development in nursing, Philadelphia, 1979, FA Davis Co.

Orem DE: Nursing: concepts of practice, New York, 1971, McGraw-Hill Book Co, Inc.

Orem DE: Nursing: concepts of practice, ed 2, New York, 1980, McGraw-Hill Book Co, Inc.

Orem DE: Nursing: concepts of practice, ed 3, New York, 1985, McGraw-Hill Book Co, Inc.

Orem DE: Nursing: concepts of practice, ed 4, St. Louis, 1991, Mosby-Year Book, Inc.

Orlando IJ: The discipline and teaching of nursing process: an evaluation study, New York, 1972, G.P. Putnam's Sons.

Orlando IJ: The dynamic nurse-patient relationship: function, process, and principles, New York, 1961, G.P. Putnam's Sons (republished in 1990 by the National League for Nursing).

Parse RR: Man-living-health: a theory of nursing, New York, 1981, John Wiley & Sons.

Parse RR: Man-living-health: a theory of nursing. In Riehl-Sisca J, editor: Conceptual models for nursing practice, ed 3, Norwalk, 1989, Appleton & Lange, pp 253–57.

Parse RR, Coyne AB, and Smith MJ: Nursing research: qualitative methods, Bowie, Md, 1985, Brady Communications Co, pp 9–13.

Parse RR: Nursing science: major paradigms, theories and critiques, Philadelphia, 1987, WB Saunders.

Paterson JG and Zderad LT: Humanistic nursing, New York, 1976, John Wiley & Sons (republished in 1987 by the National League for Nursing).

Peplau HE: The art and science of nursing: similarities, differences, and relations, *Nurs Sci Q* 9(1):8–15, 1988.

Peplau HE: Interpersonal relations in nursing, New York, 1952, GP Putnam's Sons.

Rogers ME: An introduction to the theoretical basis of nursing, Philadelphia, 1970, FA Davis Co.

Rogers ME: Nursing: a science of unitary human beings. In Riehl-Sisca J, editor: Conceptual models for nursing practice, ed 3, Norwalk, 1989, Appleton & Lange, pp 181–88.

Rogers ME: Nursing: a science of unitary man. In Riehl JP and Roy Sr C, editors: Conceptual models for nursing practice, ed 2, New York, 1980, Appleton-Century-Crofts, pp 329–37.

Rogers ME: Science of unitary human beings: a paradigm for nursing. In Clements IW and Roberts FB, editors: Family health: a theoretical approach to nursing care, New York, 1983, John Wiley & Sons, pp. 219–28.

Roy Sr C: Introduction to nursing: an adaptation model, Englewood Cliffs, 1976, Prentice-Hall, Inc.

Roy Sr. C: Introduction to nursing: an adaptation model, ed 2, Norwalk, 1984, Appleton-Century-Crofts.

Roy Sr C: The Roy adaptation model. In Riehl JP and Roy Sr C, editors: Conceptual models for nursing practice, ed 2, New York, 1980, Appleton-Century-Crofts, pp 179–88.

Roy Sr C: The Roy adaptation model. In Riehl-Sisca J, editor: Conceptual models for nursing practice, ed 3, Norwalk, 1989, Appleton & Lange, pp 105–14.

Roy Sr C and Roberts S: Theory construction in nursing: an adaptation model, Englewood Cliffs, 1981, Prentice-Hall, Inc.

Travelbee J: Interpersonal aspects of nursing, Philadelphia, 1966, FA Davis Co.

Travelbee J: Interpersonal aspects of nursing, ed 2, Philadelphia, 1971, FA Davis Co.

Watson J: New dimensions of human caring theory, *Nurs Sci Q* 9(4):175–81, 1988.

Watson J: Nursing: human science and human care, Norwalk, 1985, Appleton-Century-Crofts.

Watson J: Nursing: the philosophy and science of caring, Boston, 1979, Little, Brown & Co (republished in 1988 by the National League for Nursing).

Watson J: Watson's philosophy and theory of human caring. In Riehl-Sisca J, editor: Conceptual models for nursing practice, ed 3, Norwalk, 1989, Appleton & Lange, pp 219–36.

Wiedenbach E: Clinical nursing: a helping art, New York, 1964, Springer Publishing Co, Inc.

Appendix B

INTERPRETIVE SUMMARY:
Midrange Theories

SELECTED MIDRANGE THEORIES PROPOSING RELATIONSHIPS IN SPECIFIC AREAS OF NURSING PRACTICE: 1985–93

The summaries provided here are only a partial selection of the midrange theories now appearing in the nursing literature. These theories were selected because they illustrate the dimensions of the system for theory development that we emphasize in this text. These are not complete descriptions or critical reflections of the theorists' works. Rather, they are interpretive descriptions of the essential features of the emerging theories. They may be used as a basis for initial comparisons of theorists' works and as a basis for selecting a particular work for further description and critical reflection. A notation of the definitive theoretic writing precedes the summary.

E. T. PATTERSON AND E. S. HALE

A Theory of Menstrual Care Activities of Daily Living
Making sure: integrating menstrual care practices into activities of daily living, 1985

Focus

Report of a grounded theory study to inductively develop a substantive theory about integrating menstrual care practices into daily activities.

Concepts/Conceptual Meaning

Making sure, the core concept of the theory, is defined as the process that enables menstruating women to continue their daily activities knowing that their practices of menstrual care are effective and that the menstrual care demand can be met efficiently and effectively. Accidents are errors in making sure. Day of flow is a condition affecting making sure. Backup mechanisms are the strategies used to enhance making sure. Public and private are the contexts affecting making sure. Attending, calculating, and juggling are the sub-processes of making sure. Attending is the process of assessing the current menstrual demand. Calculating is a cognitive process of placing the menstrual care demand within the broader system of daily care demands that results in a decision about what to do with respect to menstrual self-care. Juggling is the process of assuring that time, space, and supplies coincide to meet menstrual self-care demands. The concepts of the theory are analogous to the concepts of Orem's general theory of self-care (1980).

Structure and Context of Theory

Making sure is composed of the three subprocesses of attending, calculating, and juggling. The three subprocesses occur in stages that are sequential phases of the core process of making sure; they are analogous to Orem's estimative, transitional, and productive operation of self-care (1980). Making sure occurs in the context of accidents, day of flow, back-up mechanisms, and public and private contexts. The context of the theory is that surrounding menstruating women and consists of cultural, social, and personal values regarding menstruation.

Generating and Testing the Theory

The theory was inductively generated using a grounded theory methodology. Interviews were conducted with 25 women who volunteered, or were invited to participate because of theoretically relevant variables. In addition to the interviews, informal anecdotes and serendipitous sampling were used—stories volunteered by friends and colleagues, or overhead conversations in public restrooms. The process of data analysis involved coding, memoing and sorting; ongoing comparison of incidents and codes was done to collapse categories into higher-level categories.

Deliberately Applying Theory

The purpose for developing this theory was to provide insight into nursing care that can enhance a woman's self-care ability, particularly in the early experience with menstruation. The theory has implications for education related to self-care activities, particularly with anticipating menarche and in preventing toxic shock syndrome. Further development of the theory is advocated by systematically applying the theory in practice. The authors also note that the theory may have applicability in other circumstances involving involuntary eliminative processes, such as occurs with an ostomy, urinary incontinence, or lactation.

L. R. PHILLIPS AND V. F. REMPUSHESKI

A Theory of Quality of Family Caregiving
Caring for the frail elderly at home: toward a theoretical explanation of the dynamics of poor quality family caregiving, 1986

Focus

Report of a grounded-theory approach to theory development to inductively describe dynamics of good-quality and poor-quality family caregiving, explain the relationships among contextual and perceptual variables in caring for the elderly and home, and identify points at which interventions by nurses could be effective.

Concepts/Conceptual Meaning

Five major constructs were identified. Personal identity of the elder was defined as a mental image that the caregiver has of the elder being cared for. Image of caregiving was defined as the degree to which the caregiver's personal imperatives, standards, and values are realized by the care-giving situation. Caregiver's role beliefs were defined as the standards and values held by the caregiver regarding the performance of the caregiver role, and includes the expectations for role responsibilities of the caregiver and those of the elder. Caregiver's behavioral strategies were defined as the behavior the caregiver customarily uses in responding to the elder. Perception is defined as the caregiver's interpretation of the elder's response.

Structure and Context of Theory

The five major concepts of the theory were structured as stages consistent with the framework of symbolic interactionism. Stage one, defining the process, consists of the personal identity of the elder and image of the caregiving. Stage two, cognitive processes, consists of the caregiver's role beliefs. Stage three, expressive processes, consists of the caregiver's behavioral strategies. Stage four, evaluation processes, consists of perception.

The stage one construct of personal identity of the elder involves the associated concept of reconciliation of past with present, which in turn involves six distinct processes, each of which involve three separate steps of deriving a past image, deriving a present image, and reconciling past and present using comparison. The reconciled image can be normalized or anormalized. Anormalized images can be either deified (viewing the elder as more adequate than is real) or stigmatized (viewing the elder as less adequate than is real).

The stage one construct of image of the caregiving involves the associated concept of reconciliation of proscriptions with the perceived reality of care giving, or the degree to which the caregiver's observations and perceptions of the situation diverge from the caregiver's beliefs about propriety. There are several interrelated categories of proscriptions derived in the theory development process.

The stage one constructs have a direct influence on the stage two construct of the caregiver's role beliefs, which has two associated concepts: role responsibilities of the caregiver and role responsibilities of the elder. The nature of the influence between the two stages is a major factor determining the quality of care giving.

The stage three construct, the caregiver's behavioral strategies, involves the concept of the caregiver's management strategies, or the methods used to control the elder's behavior and to resolve conflicts with the elder. Three types of management strategies were identified: positive, negative, and neutral.

The stage four construct of perception involves the concept of perception of the elder's response, or the caregiver's interpretation of the elder's role support and role enactment. This process, over time, can positively or negatively modify stage one.

Details of the structure and context of the theory are presented in diagrams and clarified using definitions and examples from the data.

Generating and Testing the Theory

The theory was inductively generated using a grounded-theory methodology. In-depth interviews were conducted with thirty-nine caregivers in two geographical locations who responded to one of two newspaper advertisements. One advertisement solicited caregivers who had a good relationship with an elder for whom they cared, and the other solicited caregivers who had an abusive or neglectful relationship with the elder. Approximately 2,000 large data bits comprised the beginning working sample, which was derived from the interviews. The data bits were subjected to constant comparative analysis, consisting of open and selective coding.

Deliberately Applying Theory

The authors state that therapeutic and cost-effective care for elders depends on the nurse's understanding of the dynamics of family caregiving and on knowing how to intervene to meet the needs of both the elder and the family members providing care. The hypotheses generated in this study provide the basis for further testing of the theory in practice, which can lead to the ability to predict caregivers who are at high risk for providing less than optimal care and to identify those points at which interventions by nurses will be most effective in high-risk care-giving situations.

M. A. WEWERS AND E. R. LENZ

A Theory of Relapse among Ex-Smokers
Relapse among ex-smokers: an example of theory derivation, 1987

Focus

Report of a theory of relapse among ex-smokers derived from a theory of recovery from alcohol abuse, and empirical testing of the derived theory using a prospective one-group-only design.

Concepts/Conceptual Meaning

Relapse is a central focus of the theory. The meaning of relapse among ex-smokers evolved from examining studies that examined the role of a specific factor in the relapse process and that examined alcohol relapse. Six factors that influence relapse were identified: sociodemographic and pretreatment smoking characteristics, nature of treatment received, and three posttreatment characteristics (stressors, coping responses, and family environment).

Structure and Context of Theory

Relapse, the central concept of the theory, was postulated to be a function of three characteristics: patient-related characteristics, treatment-related characteristics, and posttreatment characteristics. Patient-related characteristics consists of the subfactors of sociodemographic factors and pretreatment symptoms. There were no subfactors for treatment-related characteristics. Subfactors under the concept of posttreatment characteristics were stressors, coping responses, and family environment.

Patient-related characteristics of sociodemographic factors, pretreatment symptoms, and the posttreatment characteristics of stressors, coping responses, and family environment were postulated to have a major explanatory role in the theory. Because of empirical evidence that countered any differential effect of various treatment techniques, treatment-related characteristics were assigned a minor explanatory role.

The context of ex-smokers was postulated to differ from the derived context of alcohol recovery in terms of the nature of stressful life events and physiological factors arising from within the individual.

Generating and Testing the Theory

A study was conducted to examine the relationships between smoking relapse and five of the six major components of the theory using a one-group-only prospective design with 150 adults attending a smoking-cessation clinic.

Variables that operationalized the theory factors were measured prior to beginning the treatment and then three months later. The results of the study suggested that the role of posttreatment characteristics, stressors (particularly
craving), and type of coping response may be useful in designing effective treatments to prevent relapse.

Deliberately Applying Theory

The purpose underlying the development of this theory was to assist nurses in
designing effective treatments to help ex-smokers maintain long-term absti-
nence and prevent relapse. The results of this empirical test of the derived
theory suggested two major areas of focus for application of the theory. First,
symptoms of craving should be considered a high-risk predictor of relapse.
Second, a focus on problem versus emotion-focused coping responses may
improve success rates.

M. H. MISHEL

A Theory of Uncertainty
Reconceptualization of the uncertainty in illness theory, 1990

Focus

Reconceptualization of uncertainty theory (Mishel, 1988) to include experiences of living with continual uncertainty processes. Reconceptualization is
based on an examination of theory and prior empirical evidence with particular attention to the outcome portion of the theory.

Concepts/Conceptual Meaning

The original version of the uncertainty theory includes the major concept of
uncertainty, which is the inability to determine the meaning of illness because
cues necessary to assigning value are insufficient. Therefore, outcome of illness events cannot be known.

Two subconcepts identifying processes for appraisal of illness events precipitating uncertainty are identified: inference and illusion. Inference is the
construction of meaning by reference to exemplary former situations. Illusion
refers to construction of a generally positive belief system.

Two subconcepts defining outcomes of appraisal processes are identified:
danger and opportunity. For the appraisal process outcome of danger, two
coping strategies are identified: mobilizing and affect-control strategies. For
the appraisal process outcome of opportunity, the coping strategy of buffering is identified.

Adaptation, in the original version of the model, is identified as the outcome of all coping strategies, whether in response to uncertainty appraisal as danger or opportunity. Adaptation is a positive value and connotes stability and the return to equilibrium.

In the reformulated version of uncertainty theory, the concept of continual self-organization to increasing levels of complexity replaces adaptation as the outcome of uncertainty appraisal in situations of continuing and chronic uncertainty.

Structure and Context of Theory

A structure of the outcome portion of an earlier version of the uncertainty theory (Mishel, 1988) is provided. A narrative also explains and adds structure to the visual of the earlier version as well as the reformulated version of the theory. The structure is a time-ordered linear framework that begins with the situation of uncertainty in illness. Uncertainty is appraised by two processes: inference or illusion. The theory is structured so both processes are influenced by (1) the patient, (2) their social resources, and (3) health care providers. Inference, or comparison of present situations with earlier situations, can result in appraisal of uncertainty as either danger or opportunity. Illusion, or the construction of a belief system that is positive, will usually result in a view of uncertainty as opportunity. Whether appraised as danger or opportunity, coping with uncertainty follows its appraisal. If appraised as danger, coping strategies will seek to decrease uncertainty. If appraised at opportunity, coping will maintain uncertainty. Two strategies to decrease uncertainty are structured: mobilizing or affect-control strategies. Strategies to maintain uncertainty are structured to include buffering strategies.

In the earlier version of the theory, which was developed in the context of acute illness with a generally downward course, adaptation was the outcome of coping. Adaptation was assumed to be a positive state where uncertainty was successfully manipulated in the desired direction. Adaptation constituted the end point of the theory.

The original theory was structured to include cultural biases inherent in Western worldview. Assumptions reflecting this bias were identified to include (1) a temporal invariability in the appraisal of uncertainty, (2) uncertainty is generally aversive, and (3) uncertainty is a stable state rather than a process. The author states this bias is reflected in prior research findings and limits advancing the theory. The reformulation of the theory challenges these assumptions and utilizes theory derivation as described by Walker and Avant (1989).

The theory is reformulated for the context of long-term chronic uncertainty situations. In long-term illness situations, the early acute disruptions that create uncertainty and a high level of instability provide the foundation for evolving a new sense of order within the human system. Chaos theory is the perspective borrowed for reformulation of the outcome portion of the uncertainty theory. New levels of self-organization become the end point or the continuing process in response to the uncertainty of chronic illness.

The reformulation also discards the concept of illusion as a way to appraise uncertainty and the possibility of appraising uncertainty as negative, or as danger. Rather, the theory is structured so uncertainty as opportunity is the view maintained by the environmental forces of support resources and healthcare providers. There are four factors identified that block reevaluation of uncertainty and continual self-organization to higher levels of complexity. These blocks occur when (1) patients' supportive resources do not promote a probabilistic view of life, (2) the patient caretakers others, (3) the patient is isolated from social interactional contexts, and (4) providers focus on certainty and definite illness outcomes. Blocks to the continual reintegration of uncertainty to new levels of self-organization can result in posttraumatic stress syndrome.

The reconceptualization of uncertainty theory is grounded in assumptions inherent in chaos theory that characterize far-from-equilibrium systems.

Generating and Testing the Theory

The theory undergoing reconceptualization was the result of approximately ten years of ongoing empirical research and theory formulation in a variety of health and illness contexts.

The author suggests the need for empirical research for the newly reformulated theory. Also, the practical use of the theory to promote a view of the uncertainty of life and the need to create unpredictable contingencies out of seemingly unrelated situations is suggested.

Deliberately Applying Theory

The author does not specifically address research strategies for deliberative application aside from the suggested need for empirical research. Deliberative application might be accomplished through clinical application of the theory with subsequent theory reformulation based on careful analysis of the experiences of clinicians.

A. A. QUINN

A Theory of Perimenopausal Process
A theoretical model of the perimenopausal process, 1991

Focus

Qualitative study to generate theory related to women's experience of perimenopausal processes.

Concepts/Conceptual Meaning

A core variable and four subprocesses emerged from data analysis. The core variable of integrating a changing me was the central concept. Four subprocesses were identified: (1) tuning into me (my body and moods represented awareness of physical and emotional changes), (2) facing a paradox of feelings included negative and positive feelings about the menopausal experience, (3) contrasting impressions included processes of resolving conflicting information about the menopause, and (4) making adjustments referred to changes and alterations made in response to life changes. Subprocesses were further defined by narrative discussion that included examples and delineation of additional subprocesses.

Structure and Context of Theory

A theoretical structure of a pinwheel was provided. The core variable (integrating a changing me) was located at the center. The four subprocesses were integrated and linked with the core variable. The subprocesses were not depicted as sequential or linear. The subprocesses were further structured as follows. Tuning into me included processes of changing control and uncertainty in relation to qualitative and quantitative changes surrounding the menstrual cycle, hot flashes, breast tenderness, weight fluctuation, skin character, energy levels, and moods. Facing a paradox of feelings included both negative and positive feelings around getting older, reproduction, physical vulnerability, and the uncertainty of the future. Contrasting impressions were structured to include processing conflicting information about menopause acquired from stories, communication with others, exposure to media, and self-beliefs. Making adjustments included self-care practices to maintain health, coping strategies to handle stress, and caring activities. Making adjustment processes were further structured into changing diets, exercising, taking vitamins and calcium, creating time for self, making life accommodations, seeking solitude, promoting change, recognizing physical limits, putting lives in perspective, and regaining control. Further structure was provided throughout by use of examples and quotes from participants.

The theory was contextualized for the perimenopausal process as experienced by women. The structuring assumed (1) menopause was a natural process, (2) meaning attributed to the process was culturally based, (3) women's health is not synonymous with reproductive health, and (4) women's self-reports of their experience had validity.

Generating and Testing the Theory

The theory was generated using a grounded-theory methodology. Two main questions were asked: What is the process of menopause for perimenopausal women? and What are the self-care practices used for? Perimenopause was defined as the cognitive, affective, and behavioral/physical responses of women aged 40 to 60. Self-care practices were defined consistent with the self-care theory of Dorothea Orem (1980) to maintain life, health, and well-being.

Twelve women who were not on hormone therapy and who had varied backgrounds regarding marital status, education, and parity participated in the study. Women were interviewed and kept daily logs for two months. Field notes also contributed data. Theoretical sampling was used throughout data generation and analysis. Data were coded, categorized, and sorted using ethnographs to produce the core variable and related subprocesses. The truth value was established by confirming study findings with the women experiencing the perimenopausal process.

Deliberately Applying Theory

The author suggests use of the theory to understand the perimenopausal process and facilitate women's integration of the process. Providing a forum for women to express their concerns, share their stories, and receive information about the experience is cited as a clinical application of the theory. The use of the clinician's experience in applying the theory to subsequently expand and refine it could represent deliberative application processes, although this is not suggested by the author. The author does suggest further research in a variety of cultural and socioeconomic groups to broaden and expand the beginning theory.

P. G. REED

A Theory of Self-Transcendence
Toward a nursing theory of self-transcendence: deductive reformulation using developmental theories, 1991

Focus

Using deductive reformulation as method for developing theory, the author reformulated life-span developmental theory from psychology based on Rogers' general conceptual system of nursing.

Concepts/Conceptual Meaning

The definition of self-transcendence was based on reformulation that focused on areas of incongruence between life-span development theory and Rogers' conceptual system for nursing. Self-transcendence was defined as expansion of self-boundaries multidimensionally—inwardly, outwardly, and temporally. Inward expansion involves introspective experience. Outward expansion involves reaching out to others. Temporal expansion is a process whereby past and future are integrated in the present. Self-transcendence is related conceptually to well-being, particularly in terms of mental health.

Structure and Context of Theory

The structure and context of theory are expressed in two propositions that are set forth as central to the theory. These are
1. Self-transcendence is greater in persons facing end-of-own-life issues than in persons not confronted with such issues.
2. Self-transcendence is positively related to indicators of well-being in persons facing end-of-own-life issues.

Generating and Testing the Theory

The propositions of the theory were tested in five studies by Reed (1986a, 1986b, 1987, 1989, 1991) that examined spiritual and psychosocial self-transcendence. The people who participated in these studies were either terminally ill adults or were middle-old and eldest-old adults. The author developed a Spiritual Perspective Scale to measure multidimensional personal boundary expansion and a self-transcendence scale to measure psychosocial expressions of self-transcendence in later life. In addition to the quantitative analyses, qualitative data were analyzed using matrix analysis. The findings of all of the studies supported the initial propositions of the theory and provided a beginning empirical base for the theory.

Deliberately Applying Theory

The theory provides a rationale for nurses to attend to spiritual and psychosocial expressions of self-transcendence with clients who are experiencing end-of-own-life issues. The author notes that nursing therapies to help clients expand self-boundaries need to be tested in clinical practice. Potential approaches to nursing care that could be used in deliberative application include meditation, self-reflection, visualization, religious expression, peer counseling, journal keeping, and life-review processes.

K. M. SWANSON

A Theory of Caring in Perinatal Nursing
Empirical development of a middle-range theory of caring, 1991

Focus

A report of an inductively developed theory of caring derived from three perinatal contexts.

Concepts/Conceptual Meaning

Caring is a central concept. Conceptual meaning was derived from empirical (phenomenologically based) study. The meaning of caring was expressed as five caring processes, each with four to five subprocesses. A discussion of each process further clarified meaning. An empirically based definition of caring was proposed. Conceptual meaning was validated by comparison with theoretical writings of Patricia Benner (1984), Nel Noddings (1984), and Jean Watson (1985).

Structure and Context of Theory

Theory is structured in tabular form as five distinct but overlapping processes that define caring in the context of study. These five processes are (1) knowing, (2) being with, (3) doing for, (4) enabling, and (5) maintaining belief. Subdimensions that further define each process are listed. The narrative discussion and the empirically derived definition of caring provides further structure for the dimensions of caring.

The context of derivation was perinatal nursing. Three subcontexts from which the theory was structured were (1) women who recently miscarried, (2) caregivers in a newborn intensive care unit, and (3) young mothers at social risk.

Generating and Testing the Theory

The theory was generated by successive, phenomenologically based studies within separate, but related, contexts. Women who miscarried were interviewed, and the five dimensions of caring emerged. Successive studies confirmed and refined the dimensions of caring that had emerged from the initial study. The second study utilized participant observation of care providers, attendance at ethics grand rounds, and interviews with various care providers including nurses, physicians, fathers, mothers, an ethicist, a nursing administrator, and a social worker.

Deductive testing of the theory is in process. Women who have miscarried are receiving counseling grounded in the theory of caring. Outcomes related to healing and the meaning of the human experience of health and illness will be assessed.

Deliberately Applying Theory

The generation and testing operations that gave rise to the theory constituted deliberately applying theory since the initial study formed the basis for a second and third deliberative attempt to modify and strengthen the theory.

Cross-validation of the theory was provided by comparison of the emerging theory with works of Nel Noddings (1984), Patricia Benner (1984) and Jean Watson (1985).

Deliberative application is proposed for other contexts of caring to determine the generalizability of the theory. Findings suggested congruence with non-nursing theories of caring, which supports generalizability to non-nursing contexts.

J. M. HITCHCOCK AND H. S. WILSON

A Theory of Personal Risking
Personal risking: lesbian self-disclosure of sexual orientation to professional health care providers, 1992

Focus

Report of inductively developed theory of sexual identity disclosure processes of lesbians seeking traditional health care.

Concepts/Conceptual Meaning

The basic social process of personal risking is a central concept. Conceptual meaning was derived from in-depth interviews and from the assignment of meaning using grounded-theory methodology. The meaning of personal risking is expressed through a series of complex conceptual networks of subconcepts representing processes and states related to personal risking.

Personal risking is conceptually divided into two phasic processes, which are both further defined by two subprocesses. Interactional stance is also an important concept and is defined by four subconcepts. Three additional concepts modify and determine the entire personal risking process: (1) personal attributes, (2) health care context, and (3) relevancy.

Conceptual meaning is provided by narrative description and examples from participants included in the report.

The concept of fear emerged as a basic social-psychological problem that motivates the personal-risking process.

Structure and Context of Theory

The theoretical structure is derivable from the narrative. The basic social process of personal risking is a central concept. Personal risking is structured into two phases: (1) an anticipatory phase and (2) an interactional phase. The anticipatory phase is structured into two subprocesses: imagining scenarios and cognitive strategizing. Cognitive strategizing is substructured as formalizing and scouting out. Imagining scenarios is not further structured by subprocesses. Interactional stance is substructured into four concepts: (1) passive disclosure, (2) active disclosure, (3) passive nondisclosure, and (4) active nondisclosure. It also has two subprocesses: (a) scanning and (b) monitoring. Scanning occurs prior to contact with the provider. Monitoring occurs in the context of care provision.

Three additional concepts modify and determine the entire personal risking process: (1) personal attributes, (2) health care context, and (3) relevancy. These concepts overlay the entire personal-risking process. Personal attributes are structured to include the comfort level of the lesbian with sexual orientation, the relationship status of the lesbian, and the attitudes and beliefs about health care. Health care context includes provider characteristics (sexual orientation, gender, personal and professional attributes, the client's past experiences with providers) the health care environment, its location, and cues to its friendliness.

A linear structure for the major concepts is suggested in that the anticipatory phase is followed by the interactional phase. The concept of interactional stance is an outcome of the anticipatory phase and interactional stance is implemented following the scanning process of the interactional phase. The interactional stance is continuously monitored during the implementation phase with a feedback loop to interactional stance implied. The structure of the theory needs to consider stance modification (except if the stance of active disclosure has been implemented) depending on personal attributes, health care context, and relevance of disclosure.

The concept of fear emerged as a basic social-psychological problem that helped focus the structuring of the theory; fear is shared by all participants and becomes a focus for the basic social process. Thus, the resolution or management of fear becomes a focal point for theoretical organization in that the basic social process of personal risking can be organized to show how it relates to the management of fear.

The theory was contextualized in relation to the traditional health care environment processes and providers as experienced by lesbian women of a broad age range, income levels, and years of formal education. The contextual variable of relationship status was also operating in that relationship status was not controlled.

Generating and Testing the Theory

The theory was inductively generated using a grounded-theory methodology. One-time, in-depth interviews of participants were the source of data. A three-step coding process was used in data analysis. Level I codes were substantive codes that described experiences in the participants own words. Level II codes were applied to initial clusters of level I data. Level III codes were those applied to the core concepts of the theory.

Deliberately Applying Theory

This is implied in suggestions for further development, which could accrue through deliberative application of the theory or focus on the theory-development process: generation and testing of theoretical relationships. Deliberative application in different contexts: for example, geographic location and ethnicity of respondents would further define the context and provide information on generalizability of the findings. A theory-verifying approach is suggested by the authors for exploring conditions of personal attributes, health care context, and relevancy (particularly the effect each has on the personal-risking process). Deliberative application also needs to focus on the reality of health care provider attitudes toward lesbian health issues and how they affect personal-risking processes.

C. L. WIENER AND M. J. DODD

A Theory of Illness Trajectory
Coping amid uncertainty: an illness trajectory perspective, 1993

Focus

Secondary analysis of qualitative data for congruity with an extant theoretical framework of illness trajectory. A test of the validity of this theoretical framework with cancer patients by interrelating concepts of illness trajectory, coping, and uncertainty.

Concepts/Conceptual Meaning

Illness trajectory is a central concept and names the theoretical framework to be validated. The meaning of illness trajectory evolved from studies of chronically ill persons that began in the 1960s and continued through the late 1980s. Illness trajectory is defined loosely as the path of an illness course and is further defined by three major subconcepts. The course of the disease refers to an individual's life course of living with a chronic illness, which is additionally defined by three major concepts.

Other key concepts are coping and uncertainty. The meaning of coping, as a correlate of stress, is consistent with the usage in Patricia Benner's caring theory (1989). The dimensions of uncertainty evolved from extensive qualitative data analysis.

Structure and Context of Theory

The illness trajectory theory is more specifically defined as work done over the total course of the disease. There are three subconcepts or dimensions of work done: (1) the physical unfolding of the disease, (2) the total organization of work done over the course of the disease, and (3) the reciprocal consequences for family, health care professionals, and patients. The framework is undergirded by an assumption that work occurs in a social context. Subsequent research with the illness trajectory framework identified three interrelated elements around the course of a disease as a life course. These are (1) conceptions of self and (2) evolution of self over time that (3) arise directly or indirectly from the body. The theoretical structure is consistent with the expectation that these three life course concepts work together to provide structure and continuity to living. The need for coping arises when illness, such as cancer, intrudes.

The theory developed from this base and reported in this research derived from the examination of the uncertainty data in relation to temporality, body, and identity—concepts directly related to the elements of subconcepts around the life course of disease. Three major concepts evolved: uncertain temporality, uncertain body, and uncertain identity. The dimensions of uncertain temporality included: (1) loss of temporal predictability (duration, pace, frequency of recurrence), (2) sketching out and constriction of time, and (3) time as limitless. These dimensions were correlates of patient concern about the efficacy of treatment, recurrence of illness, unreliability of symptoms, and risk inherent in treatment. The dimensions of the uncertain body included: (1) body failure (activity performance, appearance, physiological function) and (2) the body's response to treatment. These dimensions correlated with patient concerns with new bodily symptoms, with having the body's resistance in jeopardy, and with what was being done with the body. The uncertain identity arises through the body and the challenges to who the patient is.

These theoretical dimensions that evolved from interrelating uncertainty with one major facet of the illness trajectory (the life course of a disease) formed a basis for examining the second major concept of the illness (work done over this life course). This resulted in the structuring of four major concepts: illness-related work, everyday work, biographical work, and uncertainty-abatement work. Illness-related work included symptom management, following the management regimen, crisis prevention and management, and diagnostic-related work. Everyday work included housekeeping and repairing, occupational work, marital, child rearing, recreation, and daily living activities. Biographical work included gathering and dispensing information, expressing concern, caring, anger, and dividing tasks. Uncertainty-abatement work included pacing, becoming a professional patient, seeking reinforcing comparisons, engaging in reviews, setting goals, covering up, finding a safe place to let down, choosing a supportive network, and taking charge.

Uncertainty is both a response to and an outcome of work and life course processes within the illness trajectory. Coping is also a response to and outcome of uncertainty. Thus, the concepts of coping, uncertainty, and illness trajectory are structurally interrelated to allow mutual, simultaneous interaction.

The theory derived from this research is contextualized for patients with an initial or ongoing cancer diagnosis who require chemotherapy and for their families.

Generating and Testing the Theory

Utilizing the borrowed theoretical framework of illness trajectory, uncertainty was examined in light of its three elements. Uncertainty data were part of a larger study of family coping and self-care during six months of a chemotherapy experience. The core variable of "tolerating the uncertainty that permeates the disease" emerged from qualitative data analysis. This research examined the work processes (that define the concept of illness trajectory) of coping in the face of uncertainty.

The uncertainty data examined were accrued from 100 interviews of a family member of a variety of patients with cancer. Each family member was interviewed three times during a six-month period of chemotherapy, either initial or repeated. The authors acknowledge that the reexamination of existing data from the perspective of grounded-theory methodology departs from its original intent. The coding paradigm was adapted to retrospective data to elicit the dimensions of uncertainty and the management processes people use to deal with cancer and its consequences.

Deliberately Applying Theory

Deliberative application is suggested in relation to theoretical sampling under different cultural conditions or among patients with different chronic illnesses. Inherent in these suggestions is sampling with patients where uncertainty has varying significance.

That health care professionals use insights to provide care suggests the possibility for intervention studies to determine if nursing care deliberately structured to manage uncertainty and facilitate coping would have reciprocal positive effects on these experiences.

REFERENCES

Benner P: From novice to expert: excellence and power in clinical nursing practice, Menlo Park, CA, 1984, Addison-Wesley.

Hitchcock JM and Wilson HS: Personal risking: lesbian self-disclosure of sexual orientation to professional health care providers, *Nurs Res* 41(3): 178–83, 1992.

Mishel MH: Reconceptualization of the uncertainty in illness theory, *Image* 22(4):256–62, 1990.

Mishel MH: Uncertainty in illness, *Image* 20(4): 225–32, 1988.

Noddings N: Caring: a feminine approach to ethics and moral education, Berkeley, 1984, University of California Press.

Orem D: Nursing: concepts of practice, ed 2, New York, 1980, McGraw-Hill Book Co.

Patterson ET and Hale ES: Making sure: integrating menstrual care practices into activities of daily living, *Adv Nurs Sci* 7(3):18–31, 1985.

Phillips LR and Rempusheski VF: Caring for the frail elderly at home: toward a theoretical explanation of the dynamics of poor quality family caregiving, *Adv Nurs Sci* 8(4):62–84, 1986.

Quinn AA: A theoretical model of the perimenopausal process, *J Nurse Midwife* 36(1):25–29, 1991.

Reed PG: Developmental resources and expression in the elderly, *Nurs Res* 35(6):368–74, 1986.

Reed PG: Mental health of older adults, *West J Nurs Res* 11:143–63,1989.

Reed PG: Religiousness among terminally ill and health adults, *Res Nurs Health* 9:35–42, 1986.

Reed PG: Self-transcendence and mental health in oldest-old adults, *Nurs Res* 40:1–7, 1991.

Reed PG: Spirituality and well-being in terminally ill hospitalized adults, *Res Nurs Health* 10:335–44, 1987.

Reed PG: Toward a nursing theory of self-transcendence: deductive reformulation using developmental theories, *Adv Nurs Sci* 13(4):64–77, 1991.

Swanson KM: Empirical development of a middle-range theory of caring, *Nurs Res* 40(3):161–66, 1991.

Walker LO and Avant KC: Strategies for theory construction in nursing, ed 2, Norwalk, 1989, Appleton-Century-Crofts.

Watson J: Nursing: human science and human care, Norwalk, 1985, Appleton-Century-Crofts.

Wewers MA and Lenz ER: Relapse among ex-smokers: an example of theory derivation, *Adv Nurs Sci* 9(2):44–53, 1987.

Wiener CL and Dodd MJ: Coping amid uncertainty: an illness trajectory perspective, *Scholar Inq Nurs Pract* 7(1):17–30, 1993.

Glossary

This glossary provides definitions for words with multiple meanings and with a particular meaning in this text. Undefined words are consistent with standard dictionary definitions. The page numbers following each entry indicate where additional information about the word may be located.

abstract concept   Mental image derived largely from indirect evidence that is not easily represented by a specific empiric indicator. The meaning of abstract concepts contained in theories can be derived from the context of the theory and often do not have the same meaning in common language. Because abstract concepts are constructed from indirect evidence, they are often interpreted differently by different people and are influenced by an individual's own perceptions and experience. (p. 58)

accessibility   Trait of theory useful for questioning, clarifying, and understanding the degree to which concepts have indicators in observable reality. (p. 133)

armchair theory   Common language term that refers to a theory constructed from mental images without the use of research methods. Armchair theory may be developed using logic and rational argument and may also imply the expression of ideas without reference to systematic processes. (p. 62)

art/act   Form in which esthetic knowing in nursing is expressed. Each art/act is unique and particular and cannot be replicated. (p. 10)

assumption   One of the structural components of theory that is taken for granted or thought to be true without systematically generated empiric evidence. Theoretic assumptions may be taken as truth because they cannot be empirically tested, as in a value statement. Assumptions may have potential for empiric testing but are taken to be true because they are consistent with a worldview or are judged to be reasonable. Assumptions may also have a degree of empiric confirmation but are designated as assumptions within theory because they do not comprise the major focus of theoretic reasoning. The term *assumption* may be used synonymously with *supposition,* as when something is taken as "truth for the sake of argument." (pp. 94, 115)

atomistic theory   Theory that deals with a narrow scope of phenomena. The term often implies, in addition, an assumption that the whole may be understood from a study of the parts. This term may be used synonymously with micro and molecular theory. (p. 121)

axiom   Type of premise used in deductive logic, often one that is not tentative, but relatively firm. Axioms as premises are used for deducing theorems, especially in mathematics. (p. 63)

choice   The fundamental purpose toward which all knowing is directed; the outcome of integration of empiric, esthetic, ethical, and personal knowledge. (pp. 6, 49)

clarity   Trait of theory useful for questioning, clarifying, and understanding the degree to which a theory is lucid and consistent of the theory. (pp. 127, 130)

components of theory   Features of theory that are useful for describing theory. Components include purpose, concepts, definitions, relationships, structure, and assumptions. (p. 106)

concept   Complex mental formulation of experience. Concepts are a major component of theory and convey the abstract ideas within the theory. (pp. 58, 79)

conceptual framework/model   Structure composed of concepts related to form a whole. Descriptive theoretic statements may be called conceptual models or frameworks. (pp. 37, 75)

conclusions   Relationship statements that are derived from premises in a deductive logic system. Conclusions are a type of proposition and may take the form of a theorem or hypothesis. (p. 64)

consensus   Process for forming understanding that emerges from the esthetic pattern of knowing. This process requires bringing to conscious awareness the diverse perspectives of others and integrating knowledge of those perspectives. Consensus and criticism interact to provide a means for understanding the meaning of esthetic knowledge. (p. 13)

consistency   Trait related to clarity. Consistency may be semantic or structural and refers to the general agreement, harmony, and compatibility of components within the theory. (pp. 129, 130)

construct   Type of highly abstract and complex concept whose reality base can only be inferred. Constructs are formed from multiple less abstract or more empiric concepts. (p. 60)

creating conceptual meaning   Theory development process of identifying, examining, and clarifying the mental images that comprise the elements, variables, or concepts within theory. (pp. 27, 80, 161)

creative dimension of knowing   Process of knowing that draws on experience and moves toward what might be in the future. (p. 6)

criteria for concepts   Essential features of a concept formed by examining conceptual meaning. Criteria are designed with reference to the purposes for which the concept is being used and should be useful to both identify and differentiate the concept from other concepts. (p. 88)

criteria for nursing diagnoses   Essential features for a specific diagnosis to be used in a given instance or situation encountered in nursing practice. (p. 163)

critical reflection   Process that addresses questions concerning the function, purposes, and value of empiric theory. (p. 126)

criticism Process for forming understanding that emerges from the esthetic pattern of knowing. Criticism is deliberate, critical, precise, and thoughtful reflection and action directed toward transformation. Consensus and criticism interact to provide a means for understanding the meaning of esthetic knowledge. (p. 13)

deduction Form of reasoning that moves from the general to the specific. In *deductive logic,* two or more premises as relational statements are used to draw a conclusion. In *deductive research processes,* an abstract theoretic relationship is used to derive specific questions or hypotheses. (p. 63)

definition Component of theory that indicates the empiric basis for a concept. Definitions are statements of meaning that provide a link between theoretic abstractions and empiric indicators. Definitions may be relatively general or specific. Theoretic definitions refer to the conceptual meaning of a term, whereas operational definitions specify how the concept is empirically assessed. (pp. 60, 92, 110)

deliberately applying the theory Theory development process for testing the usefulness of theory in practice. This process draws on research methods and places theory within the context of nursing practice to ensure that theory serves the goals of the profession. (pp. 27, 101, 164)

descriptive relationships Statements that provide an account of what something is. Descriptive relationships provide an image or impression of the nature or attributes of a phenomenon. (p. 111)

dialogue Process for forming understanding that arises from ethical knowing in nursing. Dialogue is an exchange of various points of view concerning what is right, good, or responsible. This process, in interaction with the process of justification, provides a means for challenging, rethinking, reforming, and clarifying ethical knowledge. (p. 12)

direct observation Perception of the existence of an object, property, or event by sensory means. Perception occurs at the time the phenomenon exists in reality in such a way that the object, property, or event can be objectively verified as present by more than one observer. (pp. 58, 161)

discipline Group of individuals engaged in developing a body of knowledge, the structured knowledge within an area of concern or domain of inquiry. (pp. 2, 46)

empiric-abstract continuum Means to visualize or represent the extent to which concepts have a basis in empiric reality. Empiric concepts have a direct reality basis, whereas abstract concepts have an indirect basis in empiric reality. (p. 57)

empiric concept Mental image derived from relatively direct sensory experience. A concept that represents an object, property, or event is referred to as empiric when it is experienced by the senses and can be verified and similarly described by many different observers. Empiric concepts are often more easily represented by empiric indicators than abstract concepts and can be directly observed. (p. 58)

empiric indicators Object, property, or event that is verifiable in reality; the sensory experience related to a concept. Concrete concepts have more direct empiric indicators; abstract concepts require the construction of indirect measures or tools that provides an approximate empiric measurement of some feature of the phenomenon. (pp. 58, 98, 133, 150, 161)

empirics The pattern of knowing in nursing that is the science of nursing, expressed in such forms as facts, models and scientific-empiric theories. (pp. 7–8)

empiric testing Systematic means of validating empiric reality or of observing and assessing phenomena that occur in reality. Empiric testing usually implies that research methods are used in the process of validation. (pp. 27, 99)

empiric theory Theory that expresses empiric knowledge in nursing, drawing on ideas about human science and nursing as a practice profession. (p. 20)

esthetics The pattern of knowing in nursing based on comprehension of meaning, expressed in an art/act. (pp. 10–11)

ethical principles or guidelines Statements that express the values on which actions are based. (p. 8)

ethical theory Type of theory that is developed to justify value positions. The concepts of ethical theory may be operationalized empirically, but empiric reality is not adequate for judging the validity of the theory. The adequacy of the theory is judged by the consistency of logic against the underlying value assumptions on which the theory is based. (p. 8)

ethics Pattern of knowing in nursing focusing on moral knowledge; expressed as principles and guidelines. (p. 8)

explanatory relationships Statements that provide ideas about how events happen, indicating how related factors affect or result in certain phenomena. (p. 111)

expressive dimensions of knowing Ways in which nursing's patterns of knowing are communicated and shared. Empirics and ethics are expressed in verbal forms; personal knowing and esthetics are expressed in human actions and behavior. (p. 6)

fact Objectively verifiable event, object, or property; a phenomenon that is reported similarly by more than one person. (p. 75)

general definition A statement of the meaning of a term or concept that sets forth characteristics of the phenomenon or what the phenomenon is associated with. A specific definition, by contrast, states particular characteristics, or indicators, that name what the phenomenon is. (p. 110)

generality Trait of theory that refers to the range of phenomena to which the theory applies. Generality combined with simplicity yields parsimony. (p. 132)

generalizability Extent to which research findings can be applied to or used as a basis for making decisions in like situations. Generalizability is affected by the soundness of the conceptualization process, the research design, and the analysis of the data. (p. 156)

generating and testing theoretic relationships   Theory development process that includes (1) empirically grounding emerging relationships, (2) explicating empiric indicators, and (3) validating the relationships through empiric methods.
(pp. 27, 97)

grand theory   Theory that deals with broad goals and concepts representing the total range of phenomena of concern within a discipline. This term may be used
to imply macro, molar, and holistic theory. (p. 120)

grounded theory   Theory generated from inductive research processes; the source
of data is empiric reality. (pp. 145, 153)

holism   Perspective that is based on the assumption that a whole is an emergent
and cannot be reduced to discrete elements or be analyzed without residue into
the sum of its parts. Holism may also refer to an emphasis on the value of the
whole but with consideration of discrete parts that are interrelated. (p. 46)

holistic theory   Theory that deals with a broad scope of phenomena. A theory of
high-level wellness is holistic in comparison to a theory of pain alleviation. Use
of the term *holistic theory* often implies, in addition, an assumption that the
whole is greater than the sum of its parts. This term may be used to imply macro
and grand theory. (p. 120)

hypothesis   Tentative statement of relationship between two or more variables that
can be empirically tested. The term *hypothesis* is generally used to refer to a relationship statement that is tested using specific research methods. (pp. 63, 147)

importance   Trait of theory useful for questioning, clarifying, and understanding
the extent to which a theory is clinically significant or has value for the profession. (p. 134)

indirect observation   Perception of phenomenon or methods that assess properties
or traits from which the existence of the phenomenon can be inferred.
(pp. 58, 152)

induction   Form of reasoning that moves from the specific to the general. In *inductive
logic,* a series of particulars are combined into a larger whole or set of things. In *inductive research,* particular events are observed and analyzed as a basis for formulating general theoretic statements, often called grounded theory. (p. 65)

integration   Process required for and arising from determining the credibility of all
patterns of knowing. (p. 14)

intuiting   Direct, embodied apprehension of a situation without any reasoning
process. Intuiting is part of the creative dimension of the esthetic pattern of
knowing, whereby the meaning of the moment comes from deep within the subjective experience and from the context of the individual's human experiences
and becomes expressed through in-the-moment being in the situation. (p. 10)

isolated research   Research that is completed without recognized reference or linkage to theory. (p. 140)

justification   Process for forming understanding that arises from ethical knowing in nursing; justification provides an explicit description of the values on which an ethical ideal rests and the line of reasoning toward which an ethical conclusion flows. This process, in interaction with the process of dialogue, provides a means for clarifying, reforming, rethinking, and challenging ethical knowledge. (p. 12)

knowing   Individual human processes of experiencing and comprehending self and the world in ways that can be brought to some level of conscious awareness. Not all that is comprehended in the processes of knowing can be shared or communicated. What is shared, communicated, and expressed in words or in actions becomes the knowledge of a discipline. (p. 4)

knowledge   Awareness or perception of reality acquired through insight, learning, or investigation expressed in a form that can be shared. (p. 5)

law   Relationship between variables that has been thoroughly tested and confirmed. Laws are said to be highly generalizable and are relatively certain. (p. 64)

logic   System of reasoning that deals with the form of relationships among propositions without specific regard to their content. (p. 63)

macro theory   Theory that deals with a broad scope of phenomena. This term may be used to imply grand, molar, and holistic theory. (p. 120)

meta theory   Theory about the nature of theory and the processes for its development. (p. 120)

micro theory   Theory that is relatively narrow in scope or deals with a narrow range of phenomena. This term may be used to imply atomistic and molecular theory. (p. 120)

midrange theory   Theory that deals with a relatively broad scope of phenomena but does not cover the full range of phenomena that are of concern within a discipline. A theory of pain alleviation represents a midrange theory for nursing; it is broader than a theory of neural conduction of pain stimuli but narrower than the goal of achieving high-level wellness. The phenomenon of pain is a midrange concept of concern for nursing because it is only one of many phenomena that comprise the global concern of the discipline. (pp. 52, 121)

model   General term referring to symbolic representation of perceptual phenomena in words, numbers, letters, or geometric forms. Models may provide a sense of understanding as to how theoretic relationships develop and are useful to illustrate various forms of theoretic relationships. Models can be presented as part of a theory or can be constructed to show links between related theories. Models may also be physical objects that replicate certain features of the larger object, as in a model train. (p. 75)

molar theory   Theory that deals with a broad scope of phenomena. This term may be used to imply grand, macro, and holistic theory. (p. 120)

molecular theory   Theory that is relatively narrow in scope and/or deals with a narrow range of phenomena. This term may be used to imply micro and atomistic theory. (p. 120)

nursing practice Experiences a nurse encounters in the process of caring for people. Experiences include those of the person receiving care, the nurse, others in the environment, and their interactions. (pp. 22, 108)

objectivity Assumption on which methods of science are based, in which truth is thought to exist apart from or outside of the person who knows. Based on a dualistic view of the rational mind and "out there" reality as separate. (p. 3)

operational definition Statement of meaning that indicates how a term or concept can be assessed empirically. Operational definitions are inferred from theoretic definitions. They specify the empiric indicator(s) selected for the purpose of developing research and the means of observing and measuring the indicator(s). (p. 60)

paradigm Generally accepted structure or worldview within a discipline that organizes the questions, processes, and outcomes of inquiry, including theory. (p. 76)

parsimony Relative trait of theory that incorporates degrees of both simplicity and generality. A highly parsimonious theory is one that has a broad range or generality, yet is stated in very simple terms. (p. 132)

patterns gone wild The distortion that occurs when one pattern of knowing is used without forming understanding of the pattern's meaning within the context of the whole of knowing. (p. 16)

personal knowing Pattern of knowing in nursing focused on inner experience and becoming a whole, aware self. (p. 9)

philosophy Form of disciplined inquiry for the purpose of discerning general traits of reality. (p. 74)

predictive relationships Set of statements that interrelates variables so that a specified outcome can be expected when the theory is used. (pp. 96, 112)

premises Relationship statements that are used in deductive logic as a basis for forming a conclusion. In logic, the form of the argument must be valid, regardless of how sound the premises are. Examples of types of premises include hypotheses and axioms. (p. 64)

principle Brief statement of value and/or fundamental truth that is to be followed in providing nursing care. It may also refer to principles of practice, often derived from accepted facts or theoretic propositions from other disciplines. (p. 34)

processes for forming understanding Process that provides a means for integrating the significance, background, meanings, facts, and experiences that form the whole of knowing. These processes include critical questions that are addressed and sociopolitical processes of interaction that arise from the distinct nature of each pattern of knowing in nursing. Once the processes of forming understanding are engaged, the processes make all patterns accessible and create movement between and among the processes for the other patterns of knowing. (p. 11)

processes for theory development   In a practice discipline, the processes for theory development are creating conceptual meaning, structuring and contextualizing theory, generating and testing theoretic relationships, and deliberately applying the theory. (p. 26)

profession   Vocation that requires specialized knowledge, provides a role in society that is valued, and uses some means of internal regulations of its members. (p. 46)

proposition   Statement of relationship between two or more variables. The term *proposition* is a general category that includes *postulates, premise, suppositions, axioms, conclusions, theorems,* and *hypotheses.* When a distinction in meaning is made between these various terms, the distinction reflects the form or purpose of logic used or the context in which the proposition occurs. For example, a hypothesis is generally used in the context of a research study. *Axiom* and *theorem* are used to refer to the relationship statements that are made in a particular type of deductive logic. (p. 63)

purpose   A component of theory that establishes reasons underlying a theory's development; the outcome or outcomes expected to emerge if the relationships of the theory are valid. The purpose of the theory also suggests the range of situations in which the theory is expected to apply. (p. 107)

reductionism   Philosophic stance that the whole can be partitioned and understood through generalizations made from a study of the parts. (p. 43)

reflection   Process for forming understanding that arises from personal knowing in nursing. Reflection is an inner process that requires integrating a wide range of perceptions in order to actually realize what is known within the self. Reflection interacts with response to form a process of growth in understanding the self as genuine and authentic. (p. 13)

relationships   Component of theory that refers to the interconnections between concepts. (p. 111)

relationship statements   Any statement that sets forth a connection or association between two or more phenomena. This general term is used to denote both tentative and confirmed types of statements, such as propositions, laws, axioms, and hypotheses. As a more general term, it does not imply a particular form of logic or a particular context in which the statement is used. (p. 96)

replication   Process for forming understanding that arises from empiric knowing in nursing. This process draws on methods of science to determine the extent to which an observation remains consistent from one situation or time to another. This process interacts with the process of validation to form clear and accurate understanding of empiric knowledge. (p. 12)

research   Application of systematic methods of empirics in order to develop knowledge. (pp. 75, 140)

response   Process for forming understanding that arises from personal knowing in nursing. Response is what arises from others who experience the self; it reflects or mirrors back the self of the knower. Reflection interacts with response to foster growth in understanding the self as genuine and authentic. (p. 13)

science   Knowledge, including facts and theories, generated by the use of rigorous and precise methods within an area of concern; the process of using rigorous and precise methods to generate facts and theories within an area of concern. Natural science assumes invariant laws of nature that are separate from the scientist. Human science assumes that the scientist constructs, in part, what is known. (p. 74)

simplicity   Trait of theory useful for questioning, clarifying, and understanding the degree to which a theory reduces complexity by using a minimum number of descriptive components, especially concepts, to accomplish its purpose. Simplicity implies that the theory has the fewest number of conceptual ideas in relationship that are required. Simplicity combined with generality yields parsimony. (p. 131)

social-political process   Interactive methods within each of the patterns of knowing that contribute to the integrating process of forming understanding among all knowing patterns. Processes require an individual and group interaction within the dynamic cultural, political, and social context of the times. The interactive processes are empirics—replication/validation, ethics—dialogue/justification, personal knowing—response/reflection, and esthetics—consensus/criticism. (p. 12)

specific definition   Statement of the meaning of a term or concept that names the associated object, property, or event and assigns it particular characteristics as opposed to saying what the concept is like or associated with in reality. (p. 110)

structure   A component of theory that refers to the overall morphologic arrangement of specific elements, especially concepts, within the theory. (p. 112)

structuring and contextualizing theory   Theory development process of organizing relationships between and among concepts in a unique, creative, rigorous, and systematic way, consistent with the purposes of the theory. This process also includes identifying the domain, realm, or context of the theory; stating the assumptions on which the theory is based; and providing conceptual definitions of terms that guide decisions about the empiric events to which concepts relate. (pp. 27, 91)

theorem   Conclusion that is drawn from axioms as premises in a deductive form of logic. Theorems and axioms are used within the logical systems of mathematics, and the relationships expressed imply some degree of certainty or validity. (p. 65)

theoretic definition   Statement of meaning that conveys essential features of a concept in a manner that fits meaningfully within the theory. A theoretic definition specifies conceptual meaning and implies empiric indicators for concepts. This word may be used synonymously with conceptual definition. (p. 94)

theoretic framework/model   Structure comprised of concepts related in some way to form a whole. The term *theoretic framework* or *model* often connotes less tentativeness than *conceptual framework* or *model*, but often *theoretic* and *conceptual model* and *framework* are used interchangeably. (p. 75)

theory   Creative and rigorous structuring of ideas that project a tentative, purposeful, and systematic view of phenomena. (p. 71)

theory-linked research   Research that is designed with reference or linkage to theory. Theory-linked research may be theory-testing or theory-generating. Theory-
testing research ascertains how accurately existing theoretic relationships depict
reality-based events. Theory-generating research is designed to discover and describe relationships by observing empiric reality and then constructing theory
based on empiric data observed. (p. 140)

validation   Process for forming understanding that arises from empiric knowing in
nursing. Validation is a process that focuses on the accuracy of conceptual
meanings in terms of empiric evidence. Validation and replication interact to
provide a means of forming clear and accurate understandings of empiric
knowledge. (p. 12)

Bibliography

Abdellah FG: The nature of nursing science, *Nurs Res* 18(5):390–93, 1969.

Abdellah FG et al: Patient-centered approaches to nursing, New York, 1960, The Macmillan Co.

Allan JD and Hall BA: Challenging the focus on technology: a critique of the medical model in a changing health care system, *Adv Nurs Sci* 10(3):22–34, 1988.

Allen D: Nursing research and social control: alternative models of science that emphasize understanding and emancipation, *J Nurs Scholarship* 17(2):59–64, 1985.

Allen MN and Jensen L: Hermeneutical inquiry: meaning and scope, *West J Nurs Res* 12(2):241–53, 1990.

Ashley JA: Foundations for scholarship: historical research in nursing, *Adv Nurs Sci* (1):25–36, 1978.

Barzun J and Graff HF: The modern researcher, ed 4, New York, 1985, Harcourt Brace.

Beckstand J: A critique of several conceptions of practice theory in nursing, *Res Nurs Health* 3(2):69–79, 1980.

Benner P: From novice to expert: excellence and power in clinical nursing practice, Menlo Park, 1984, Addison-Wesley.

Benner P: Quality of life: a phenomenological perspective on explanation, prediction, and understanding in nursing science, *Adv Nurs Sci* 8(1):1–14, 1985.

Benner P and Wrubel J: The primacy of caring, Menlo Park, 1989, Addison-Wesley.

Benoliel JA: The interaction between theory and research, *Nurs Outlook* 25(2):108–13, 1977.

Berthold JS: Theoretical and empirical clarification of concepts, *Adv Nurs Sci* 2(5):406–22, 1964.

Berthold JS: Symposium on theory development in nursing: prologue, *Nurs Res* 17(3):196–97, 1968.

Bishop AH and Scudder JR: Nursing: the practice of caring, New York, 1991, National League for Nursing.

Bleicher J: Contemporary hermeneutics: hermeneutics as method, philosophy and critique, Boston, 1980, Routledge and Kegan Paul.

Bok S: Lying: moral choice in public and private life, New York, 1978, Pantheon Books.

Bottorff JL: Nursing: a practical science of caring, *Adv Nurs Sci* 14(1):26–39, 1991.

Boulding KE: The image, Ann Arbor, 1961, University of Michigan Press.

Butterfield PG: Thinking upstream: nurturing a conceptual understanding of the societal context of health behavior, *Adv Nurs Sci* 12(2):1–8, 1990.

Campbell JC and Bunting S: Voices and paradigms: perspectives on critical and feminist theory in nursing, *Adv Nurs Sci* 13(3):1–15, 1991.

Carper BA: Fundamental patterns of knowing in nursing, *Adv Nurs Sci* 1(1):13–23, 1978.

Carper BA: The ethics of caring, *Adv Nurs Sci* 1(3):11–19, 1979.

Chinn PL, editor: Advances in nursing theory development, Rockville, MD, 1983, Aspen Systems Corp.

Chinn PL: Debunking myths in nursing theory and research, *J Nurs Scholarship* 17(2):45–49, 1985.

Chinn PL: The art of criticism (editorial), *Adv Nurs Sci* 7(4):vii–viii, 1985.

Chinn PL: Nursing research methodology, Rockville, MD, 1986, Aspen Systems Corp.

Chinn PL: Nursing patterns of knowing and feminist thought, *Nurs Health Care* 19(2):71-75, 1989.

Chinn PL (ed.): Anthology on caring, New York, 1991, National League for Nursing.

Chinn PL and Jacobs MK: A model for theory development in nursing, *Adv Nurs Sci* 1(1):1–11, 1978.

Chinn PL and Watson MJ (ed.) Art and aesthetics in nursing, New York, 1994, National League for Nursing.

Chinn PL and Wheeler CE: Feminism and nursing, *Nurs Outlook* 33(2): 74–77, 1985.

Coppa DF: Chaos theory suggests a new paradigm for nursing science, *J Adv Nurs* 18(6): 985–91, 1993.

Coward DD: Critical multiplism: a research strategy for nursing science, *J Nurs Scholarship* 22(3):163–67, 1990.

Curtin LL: The nurse as advocate: a philosophical foundation for nursing, *Adv Nurs Sci* 1(3):1–10, 1979.

DeGroot HA: Scientific inquiry in nursing: a model for a new age, *Adv Nurs Sci* 10(3):1–21, 1988.

Dickoff J and James P: A theory of theories: a position paper, *Nurs Res* 17(3):197–203, 1968.

Dickoff J and James P: Clarity to what end? *Nurs Res* 20(6):499–502, 1971.

Dickoff J and James P: Organization and expansion of knowledge: toward a constructive assault on the imperious distinction of pure from applied knowledge, of knowledge from technology, *Dent Hyg* 62(1):15–20, 1988.

Dickoff J, James P, and Wiedenbach E: Theory in a practice discipline. Part I: Practice-oriented theory, *Nurs Res* 17(5):415–35, 1968.

Doering L: Power and knowledge in nursing: a feminist poststructuralist view, *Adv Nurs Sci* 14(4):24–33, 1992.

Donaldson SK and Crowley DM: The discipline of nursing, *Nurs Outlook* 26(2):113–20, 1968.

Dzurec LC: The necessity for and evolution of multiple paradigms for nursing research: a poststructuralist perspective, *Adv Nurs Sci* 11(4):69–77, 1989.

Dzurec LC and Abraham IL: The nature of inquiry: linking quantitative and qualitative research, *Adv Nurs Sci* 16(1):73–79, 1993.

Ellis R: Characteristics of significant theories, *Nurs Res* 17(3):217–22, 1968.

Ellis R: The practitioner as theorist, *Am J Nurs* 69(7):1434–38, 1969.

Ellis R: Commentary on ``Toward a clearer understanding of the concept of nursing theory," *Nurs Res* 20(6):493–94, 1971.

Fawcett J: The relationship between theory and research: a double helix, *Adv Nurs Sci* 1(1):49–62, 1978.

Fawcett J: Analysis and evaluation of conceptual models of nursing, ed 3, Norwalk, 1993, Appleton & Lange.

Feinstein AR: Clinical judgment, Hudington, NY, 1967, Robert E. Kreiger Publishing Co, Inc.

Fitzpatrick J and Whall A, editors: Conceptual models of nursing: analysis and application, ed 2, Norwalk, 1989, Appleton & Lange.

Flaskerud JH and Halloran EJ: Areas of agreement in nursing theory development, *Adv Nurs Sci* 3(1):1–7, 1980.

Fry ST: Toward a theory of nursing ethics, *Adv Nurs Sci* 11(2):9–22, 1989.

Fulton JS: Virginia Henderson: theorist,prophet, poet, *Adv Nurs Sci*, 10(1):1–9, 1987.

George J, editor: Nursing theories: the basis for professional practice, ed 3, Norwalk, 1990, Appleton & Lange.

Gilligan C: In a different voice: psychological theory and women's development, Cambridge, 1982, Harvard University Press.

Giorgi A: Psychology as a human science: a phenomenologically based approach, New York, 1970, Harper & Row.

Glaser B and Strauss A: The discovery of grounded theory, Chicago, 1967, Aldine Publishing Co.

Gortner SR: The history and philosophy of nursing science and research, *Adv Nurs Sci* 5(2):1–8, 1983.

Greene JA: Science, nursing and nursing science: a conceptual analysis, *Adv Nurs Sci* 2(1):57–64, 1979.

Griffin AP: Philosophy and nursing, *J Adv Nurs* 5(3):261–72, 1980.

Hagan KL: Internal affairs: a journalkeeping workbook for self-intimacy, New York, 1990, Harper & Row.

Hall LE: A center of nursing, *Nurs Outlook* 11(11):805–6, 1963.

Hall LE: Another view of nursing care and quality. In Straub KM and Parker KS, editors: Continuity in patient care: the role of nursing, Washington DC, 1966, Catholic University Press, pp 47–60.

Hardy ME, editor: Theoretical foundations for nursing, New York, 1973, MSS Information Corp.

Henderson V: The nature of nursing, New York, 1966, The Macmillan Co.

Henderson V: The nature of nursing: a definition and its implications for practice, research and education: reflections after 25 years, New York, 1991, National League for Nursing.

Hinshaw AS: Theoretical substruction: an assessment process, *West J Nurs Res* 1(4):319–24, 1979.

Hoffman AL and Bertrus PA: Theory and practice: bridging scientists and practitioners' roles, *Arch Psychiatr Nurs* 6(10):2–9, 1992.

Holmes CA: The drama of nursing, *J Adv Nurs* 17(8):941–50, 1992.

Jacobs MK: Can nursing theory be tested? In Chinn PL, editor: Methodological issues in nursing, Rockville, MD, 1986, Aspen Publishers.

Jacobs-Kramer MK and Chinn PL: Perspectives on knowing: a model of nursing knowledge, *Scholarly Inquiry Nurs Pract* 2(2):129–39,1988.

Jacobs MK and Huether SE: Nursing science: the theory-practice linkage, *Adv Nurs Sci* 1(1):63–73, 1978.

Jacox A: Theory construction in nursing: an overview, *Nurs Res* 23(1): 4–13, 1974.

Jennings BM and Meleis AI: Nursing theory and administrative practice: agenda for the 1990s, *Adv Nurs Sci* 10(3):56–69, 1988.

Johnson DE: Theory in nursing: borrowed and unique, *Nurs Res* 17(3):206–9, 1968.

Johnson DE: The behavioral system model for nursing. In Riehl JP and Roy Sr C, editors: Conceptual models for nursing practice, ed 2, New York, 1980, Appleton-Century-Crofts, pp 207–16.

Johnson DE: Some thoughts on nursing, *Clin Nurs Spec* 1(2):1–4, 1989.

Kaplan A: The conduct of inquiry, New York, 1964, Thomas Y. Crowell Co, Inc.

King IM: A theory of nursing: systems, concepts, process, New York, 1981, John Wiley & Sons.

King IM: King's general systems framework and theory. In Riehl-Sisca J, editor: Conceptual models for nursing practice, ed 3, Norwalk, 1989, Appleton & Lange, pp 149–58.

King IM: King's theory of goal attainment, *Nurs Sci Q* 5(1):19–26, 1992.

Kramer MK: Holistic nursing: implications for knowledge development and utilization. In Chaska NL, editor: The nursing profession: turning points, St. Louis, 1990, Mosby-Year Book, Inc, pp 245–54.

Kleffel D: Rethinking the environment as a domain of nursing knowledge, *Adv Nurs Sci* 14(10):40–51, 1991.

Krieger D: Foundations for holistic health nursing practices: the renaissance nurse, Philadelphia, 1981, JB Lippincott Co.

Krueter FR: What is good nursing care? *Nurs Outlook* 5(5):302–4, 1957.

Kuhn T: The structure of scientific revolutions, Chicago, 1972, The University of Chicago Press.

Laudan L: Progress and its problems, Berkeley, 1977, University of California Press.

Leddy S and Pepper JM: Conceptual bases of professional nursing, ed 3, Philadelphia, 1993, JB Lippincott Co.

Leininger MM: Transcultural nursing: concepts, theories, and practices, New York, 1978, John Wiley & Sons.

Leininger MM (ed.): Care: the essence of nursing and health, Thorofare, NJ, 1984, Charles B Slack, Inc.

Leininger MM: Leininger's theory of nursing; cultural care diversity and universality, *Nurs Sci Q* 1(4):152–60, 1988.

Leonard VW: A Heideggerian phenomenologic perspective on the concept of the person, *Adv Nurs Sci* 11(4):40–55, 1989.

Levine ME: The four conservation principles of nursing, *Nurs Forum* 6(1):45–59, 1967.

Levine ME: Introduction to clinical nursing, ed 2, Philadelphia, 1973, FA Davis Co.

Levine ME: The conservation principles: twenty years later. In Riehl-Sisca J, editor: Conceptual models for nursing practice, ed 3, Norwalk, 1989, Appleton & Lange, pp 325–37.

Lowenberg JS: Interpretive research methodology: Broadening the dialogue, *Adv Nurs Sci* 16(2):57–69, 1993.

MacPherson KI: Feminist methods: a new paradigm for nursing research, *Adv Nurs Sci* 5(2):17–26, 1983.

Malinski VM: Explorations on Martha Rogers: science of unitary human beings, Norwalk, 1986, Appleton-Century-Crofts.

Marriner-Tomey A, editor: Nursing theorists and their work, ed 3, St. Louis, 1994, Mosby-Year Book, Inc.

McKay RP: Theories, models and systems for nursing, *Nurs Res* 18(5):393–99, 1969.

Meleis, AI: Revisions in knowledge development: a passion for substance, *Scholarly Inquiry Nurs Pract* 1(1):5–19, 1987.

Meleis AI: Theoretical nursing, ed 2, Philadelphia, 1991, JB Lippincott Co.

Meleis AI: Directions for nursing theory development in the 21st century, *Nurs Sci Q* 5(3):112–17, 1992.

Melosh B: The physician's hand: work culture and conflict in American nursing, Philadelphia, 1982, Temple University Press.

Merton RK: The sociology of science: theoretical and empirical investigations, Chicago, 1973, The University of Chicago Press.

Moccia PA: A further investigation of "dialectical thinking as a means of understanding systems-in-development: relevance to Roger's principles," *Adv Nurs Sci* 7(4):33–38, 1985.

Moccia PA, editor: New approaches to theory development, New York, 1986, National League for Nursing.

Moccia PA: A critique of compromise: beyond the methods debate, *Adv Nurs Sci* 10(4):1–9, 1988.

Morse JM, editor: Critical issues in qualitative research methods, Thousand Oaks, CA, 1993, Sage Publications, Inc.

Muller ME and Dzurec LC: The power of the name, *Adv Nurs Sci* 15(3): 15–22, 1993.

Munhall PL: Nursing philosophy and nursing research: in apposition or opposition? *Nurs Res* 31(3):176–77, 1982.

Munhall PL: Methodological fallacies: a critical self-appraisal, *Adv Nurs Sci* 5(4):41–50, 1983.

Munhall PL: Methodological issues in nursing research: beyond a wax apple, *Adv Nurs Sci* 8(3):1–5, 1989.

Murphy JF: Theoretical issues in professional nursing, New York, 1971, Appleton-Century-Crofts.

Neil RM and Watts R, editors: Caring and nursing: explorations in feminist perspectives, New York, 1990, National League for Nursing.

Neuman B: The Neuman systems model, ed 2, Norwalk, 1989, Appleton & Lange.

Newman MA: Health as expanding consciousness, St. Louis, 1986, Mosby-Year Book, Inc.

Newman MA: Shifting to higher consciousness. In Parker ME, editor: Nursing theories in practice, New York, 1990, National League for Nursing, pp. 129–39.

Nicoll, LH, editor: Perspectives on nursing theory, ed 1, 1986, Little-Brown.

Nicoll LH, editor: Perspectives on nursing theory, ed 2, Philadelphia, 1992, Lippincott & Co.

Nightingale F: Notes on nursing: what it is and what it is not, New York, 1969, Dover Publications (unabridged republication of the first American edition, as published in 1860 by D. Appleton & Co.).

Noddings N: Caring: a feminine approach to ethics and moral education, Berkeley, 1984, University of California Press.

Norris CM, editor: Proceedings of the first, second and third nursing conferences, Kansas City, KS, 1969–70, University of Kansas Medical Center Department of Nursing Education.

Norris CM: Concept clarification in nursing, Rockville, MD, 1982, Aspen Systems Corp.

Nursing theories at work, Videotape, New York, National League for Nursing.

Nursing theory: a circle of knowledge, Parts I and II, Videotape, New York, National League for Nursing.

Omery A: Phenomenology: a method for nursing research, *Adv Nurs Sci* 5(2):49–64, 1983.

Orem D: Nursing: concepts of practice, ed 4, St. Louis, 1991, Mosby-Year Book, Inc.

Orlando IJ: The dynamic nurse-patient relationship: function, process, and principles, New York, 1961, GP Putnam's Sons (republished in 1990 by the National League for Nursing).

Orlando IJ: The discipline and teaching of nursing process: an evaluation study, New York, 1972, GP Putnam's Sons.

Parker ME, editor: Nursing theories in practice, New York, 1990, National League for Nursing.

Parker ME, editor: Patterns of nursing theories in practice, New York, 1993, National League for Nursing.

Parse RR: Nursing science: major paradigms, theories and critiques, Philadelphia, 1987, WB Saunders.

Parse RR: Man-living-health: a theory of nursing. In Riehl-Sisca J, editor: Conceptual models for nursing practice, ed 3, Norwalk, 1989, Appleton & Lange, pp 253–57.

Parse RR: Human becoming: Parse's theory of nursing, *Nurs Sci Q* 5(1):35–42, 1992.

Parse RR: Parse's human becoming theory: its research and practice implications. In Parker ME, editor: Patterns of nursing theories in practice, New York, 1993, National League for Nursing, pp 49–61.

Paterson JG: From a philosophy of clinical nursing to a method of nursology, *Nurs Res* 29(2):143–46, 1971 (republished in 1987 by the National League for Nursing).

Paterson JG and Zderad LT: Humanistic nursing, New York, 1976, John Wiley & Sons (republished in 1987 by the National League for Nursing).

Peplau HE: Interpersonal relations in nursing, New York, 1952, GP Putnam's Sons.

Peplau HE: The art and science of nursing: similarities, differences, and relations, *Nurs Sci Q* 1(1):8–15, 1988.

Peplau HE: Interpersonal relations in nursing: a conceptual frame of reference for psychodynamic nursing, New York, 1991, Springer Publishing Co.

Peplau HE: Interpersonal relations: a theoretical framework for application in nursing practice, *Nurs Sci Q* 5(1):13–18, 1992.

Polkinghorne D: Methodology for the human sciences, Albany, 1983, SUNY Press.

Popper KR: Conjectures and refutations: the growth of scientific knowledge, New York, 1965, Basic Books.

Quint JC: The case for theories generated from empirical data, *Nurs Res* 16(2):109–14, 1967.

Ramos MC: Adopting an evolutionary lens: an optimistic approach to discovering strength in nursing, *Adv Nurs Sci* 10(1):19–26, 1983.

Reed PG: Nursing theorizing as an ethical endeavor, *Adv Nurs Sci* 11(3):1–10, 1989.

Reichenbach H: The rise of scientific philosophy, Berkeley, 1951, University of California Press.

Reverby SM: Ordered to care: the dilemma of American nursing, 1850–1945, New York, 1987, Cambridge University Press.

Reynolds CL and Leininger MM: Cultural care diversity and universality theory, Thousand Oaks, CA, 1993, Sage Publications, Inc.

Reynolds PD: A primer in theory construction, Indianapolis, 1971, The Bobbs-Merrill Co, Inc.

Riehl-Sisca JP, editor: Conceptual models for nursing practice, ed 3, Norwalk, 1989, Appleton & Lange.

Roberts H, editor: Doing feminist research, Boston, 1981, Routledge and Kegan Paul.

Roberts SJ: Oppressed group behavior: implications for nursing, *Adv Nurs Sci* 5(4):21–30, 1983.

Rogers ME: Reveille in nursing, Philadelphia, 1964, FA Davis Co.

Rogers ME: An introduction to the theoretical basis of nursing, Philadelphia, 1970, FA Davis Co.

Rogers ME: Nursing: a science of unitary human beings. In Riehl-Sisca J, editor: Conceptual models for nursing practice, ed 3, Norwalk, 1989, Appleton & Lange.

Rogers ME: Nursing science and the space age, *Nurs Sci Q* 5(1):27–34, 1992.

Roy Sr C: Introduction to nursing: an adaptation model, ed 2, Norwalk, 1984, Appleton-Century-Crofts.

Roy Sr C: The Roy adaptation model. In Riehl-Sisca J, editor: Conceptual models for nursing practice, ed 3, Norwalk, 1989, Appleton & Lange, pp 105–14.

Roy Sr C and Andrews H: The Roy adaptation model: The definitive statement, Norwalk, 1991, Appleton & Lange.

Roy Sr C and Roberts S: Theory construction in nursing: an adaptation model, Englewood Cliffs, 1981, Prentice-Hall, Inc.

Sandelowski M: The problem of rigor in qualitative research, *Adv Nurs Sci* 8(3):27–37, 1986.

Sarter B: Evolutionary idealism: a philosophical foundation for holistic nursing theory, *Adv Nurs Sci* 9(2):1–9, 1987.

Sarter B, editor: Paths to knowledge: innovative research methods for nursing, New York, 1989, National League for Nursing.

Schlotfeldt RM: Nursing research: reflection of values, *Nurs Res* 26(1):4–9, 1977.

Schlotfeldt RM: Nursing in the future, *Nurs Outlook* 29(5):295–301, 1981.

Schultz PR and Meleis AI: Nursing epistemology: traditions, insights, questions, *J Nurs Scholarship* 20(4):217–24, 1988.

Schumacher KL and Gortner SR: (Mis)conceptions and reconceptions about traditional science, *Adv Nurs Sci* 14(4):1–11, 1992.

Silva MC: Research testing nursing theory: state of the art, *Adv Nurs Sci* 9(1):1–11, 1986.

Silva MC and Sorrell JM: Testing of nursing theory: critique and philosophical expansion, *Adv Nurs Sci* 14(4):12–23, 1992.

Smith JA: The idea of health: implications for the nursing professional, New York, 1983, Teachers College Press.

Smith MJ: Enhancing esthetic knowledge: a teaching strategy, *Adv Nurs Sci* 14(3):52–59, 1992.

Spender D: Manmade language, 2nd ed., Boston, 1985, Routledge and Kegan Paul.

Stern PN: Grounded theory methodology: its uses and processes, *J Nurs Scholarship* 12(1):20–23, 1980.

Stevens-Barnum BJ: Nursing theory: analysis and evaluation, ed 4, Philadelphia, 1994, JB Lippincott.

Stevens BJ: Nursing theories: one or many? In Grace HK and McCloskey JC, editors: Current issues in nursing, Boston, 1981, Blackwell Scientific Publications, pp 35–43.

Stevens PE: A critical social reconceptualization of environment in nursing: implications for methodology, *Adv Nurs Sci* 11(4):56–68, 1989.

Theory development: What? Why? How? New York, 1978, National League for Nursing.

Thompson JL: Practical discourse in nursing: going beyond empiricism and historicism, *Adv Nurs Sci* 7(4):59–71, 1985.

Thompson JL: Critical scholarship: the critique of domination in nursing, *Adv Nurs Sci* 19(1):27–38, 1987.

Tong R: Feminist thought: a comprehensive introduction, Boulder and San Francisco, 1989, Westview Press.

Travelbee J: Interpersonal aspects of nursing, Philadelphia, 1966, FA Davis Co.

Travelbee J: Interpersonal aspects of nursing, ed 2, Philadelphia, 1971, FA Davis Co.

Twomey JG, Jr: Analysis of the claim to distinct nursing ethics: normative and non-normative approaches, *Adv Nurs Sci* 11(3):25–32, 1989.

Walker LO and Avant KC: Strategies for theory construction in nursing, ed 2, Norwalk, 1988, Appleton & Lange.

Watson J: Nursing: human science and human care, Norwalk, 1985, Appleton-Century-Crofts.

Watson J: New dimensions of human caring theory, *Nurs Sci Q* 1(4):175–81, 1988.

Watson J: Nursing: the philosophy and science of caring, Boston, 1979, Little, Brown & Co (republished in 1988 by the National League for Nursing).

Watson J: Watson's philosophy and theory of human caring. In Riehl-Sisca J, editor: Conceptual models for nursing practice, ed 3, Norwalk, 1989, Appleton & Lange, pp 219–36.

Watson J: Transpersonal caring: a transcendent view of person, health and nursing. In Parker ME, editor: Patterns of nursing theories in practice, New York, 1993, National League for Nursing, pp 277–88.

Wheeler CE and Chinn PL: Peace and power: a handbook of feminist process, ed 3, New York, 1991, National League for Nursing.

Wiedenbach E: Clinical nursing: a helping art, New York, 1964, Springer Publishing Co, Inc.

Williams DM: Political theory and individualistic health promotion, *Adv Nurs Sci* 12(1):14–25, 1989.

Wilson J: Thinking with concepts, London, 1963, Cambridge University Press.

Winstead-Fry P: The scientific method and its impact on holistic health, *Adv Nurs Sci* 2(4):1–7, 1980.

Winstead-Fry P, editor: Case studies in nursing theory, New York, 1986, National League for Nursing.

Yeo M: Integration of nursing theory and nursing ethics, *Adv Nurs Sci* 11(3):33–42, 1989.

Index

specific, 219
theoretic, 219
of theory; *see* Theory, definition of
Deliberative application of theory, 101–102, 213
Description
in empirics, 7–8
of theory, 105–123; *see also* Theory, description of
Descriptive relationships, 213
Development
of research 146–156; *see also* Research, development of theory, 77–103; *see also* Theory development
Diagnosis, nursing, 163–164
Dialogue, 213
understanding and, 14
Dickoff and James' definition of theory development, 39, 68–70
Differentiation
of similar concepts, 162
structural idea form of, 113, 114
Dimensions of knowing, 6
creative, 6, 212
expressive, 214
Direct observation, 213
Direction in theory, evolving, 50–53
Discipline, 213
nursing as, 46–47
of nursing process, 173
Discrete components, structural idea form of, 114
Diversity, cultural care, 184–185
Dock's contributions to nursing theory development, 35
Dynamic nurse-patient relationships, 173–174

E

Early nursing models, 40–46
health in, 43–44
nature of nursing in, 41
person in, 43
society and environment in, 43
Education, nursing theory development and, 38
Ego as concept, 60
Ellis' definition of theory, 71
Emergence of theory, 31–53; *see also* Theory, emergence of
Emerging relationships, empirically grounded, 97–98
Empathy, 163
Empiric abstract continuum, 59, 213

Empiric concepts, 213; *see also* Empirics
abstract concept and, 58–62
Empiric indicators, 213; *see also* Empirics
naming, 98–99
identification of, 161–162
Empiric testing, 214
Empiric theory, 214
Empirically grounded emerging relationships, 97–98
Empirics, 7–8, 214
knowing and, 7–8
nursing theory as expression of, 19–30
creation of, 26–30
definition in, 20
development processes for, 30
uses of, 21–26
patterns gone wild and, 16
Engaging in esthetics, 10–11
Environment
in early nursing models, 43, 45
man and, 188–189
relationship of individual to, 115
Esthetics, 10–11, 214
engaging in, 10–11
knowing and, 10–11
patterns gone wild and, 16–18
Ethical theory, 214
Ethics, 8–9, 214
knowing and, 8–9
patterns gone wild and, 16–18
principles of, 214
in theory-linked research, 143
Evidence in determining theory usefulness, 164–168
Experience, 78
Explanations
in determining theory usefulness, 166,
in empirics, 7–8
Explanatory relationships, 214
Expression of knowledge, 4–7
Expressive dimensions of knowing, 6, 214

F

Fact, 75, 214
Features of theory, definitions and, 73–76
Field observation, 145
Form, structural; *see* Structure
Formal methods of study, 102
Format, 63–64
Foundational to dependent structural idea form, 114
Framework
conceptual, 212
theoretic, 219